D0319300

the
STEP
COUNTER
diet

If your step counter is in any way faulty, please return it to the address below and we will of course replace the product.

Thorsons

HarperCollins*Publishers*

77–85 Fulham Palace Road

Hammersmith

London

W6 8JB

Joanna Hall MSc

the
STEP
COUNTER
diet

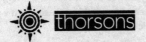

thorsons

Thorsons
An Imprint of HarperCollins*Publishers*
77–85 Fulham Palace Road,
Hammersmith, London W6 8JB

The website address is: www.thorsonselement.com

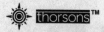

and *Thorsons* are trademarks of
HarperCollins*Publishers* Ltd

First published by Thorsons 2004

2

© Joanna Hall 2004

Joanna Hall asserts the moral right to be
identified as the author of this work

A catalogue record of this book is
available from the British Library

ISBN 0 00 720251 2

Printed and bound in Great Britain by
Clays Ltd, St Ives plc

All rights reserved. No part of this publication may be
reproduced, stored in a retrieval system, or transmitted,
in any form or by any means, electronic, mechanical,
photocopying, recording or otherwise, without the prior
written permission of the publishers.

Contents

Introduction

Hello, and welcome to my Step Counter Diet!

This is just about the most simple yet effective diet plan you will ever find. All you need to do is put one foot in front of another and walk! Combine it with my eating principles and in 28 days you will have a slimmer, fitter body and you will enjoy loads more energy. It has delivered fantastic results for hundreds of my clients, and I know it will work for you too!

You will find the Step Counter Diet easy to follow and the day by day charts help you stay on track and provide that on-going motivation.

Not only is the Step Counter Diet easy, but just about anyone can do it and feel the benefits – young, old, fit and unfit. So what are you waiting for?

Let's get going!

Be active,

Joanna

What will the plan do for me?

Everyone who has completed this programme has lost inches and felt fantastic. If you stick with it, you will be just as successful – I promise!

You will lose weight
You will lose inches
You will feel more energetic
You will be fitter
You will feel back in control
You could benefit from lowering elevated cholesterol levels
You could enjoy better sleep...

...and many have reported having better sex!

So how does the Step Counter Diet work?

SECTION 1

how the plan works

This plan is about getting results by fitting exercise and healthy eating into the life *you* lead. It is a focused eating and walking plan designed to help you lose weight and inches – especially around your middle and waistline.

The eating plan follows easily implemented principles, based on my Carb Curfew concept. I'll talk more about these principles on page 18. You'll soon see how they work and how easily they can be slotted into your life.

The exercise plan is based on walking and just five tummy exercises. That's it. You don't need a gym membership, expensive exercise kit or flashy trainers – just a pair of comfortable walking shoes, your free pedometer and enough space on the floor to do some tummy exercises. And absolutely anyone can do it – I promise you.

The plan runs over 28 days and you can either follow the 28-day plan as strictly as you want or follow a more relaxed weekly approach, depending on what suits you. You'll find lots of tips throughout the book, so you need not feel alone. Don't forget, you'll also find lots of advice on the Q&A section of my website: www.joannahall.com

Being successful does require a little prior preparation, so in this section I'll outline how the plan works and how to get yourself ready in the days leading up to the start. The easy-to-follow 5-day countdown not only helps you get organised before your 28 days to success but also gets you into that all-important positive mindset. In my experience, getting yourself in the right headspace can be a deciding factor to your success. You may also want to look at my book *Drop a Size for Life* as this contains my 7-step approach to getting you mentally prepared.

So if you are ready let's:

Plan Ahead!
Be Prepared!
Become Empowered!

Recording your progress

Recording your measurements is an important part of tracking your progress. Body Mass Index (BMI) is one way to define obesity, using the relationship between your height and weight. To calculate your BMI divide your weight in kilograms by your height in metres squared. You'll find an automatic BMI calculator on my web site www.joannahall.com. A BMI value of 30 is indicative of being obese, a BMI value of 40 and above is indicative of being morbidly obese and a BMI of 25 is indicative of being overweight.

But while BMI is widely recognised as a measure of obesity it does not give a strong indication of your health risks as it does not account for your levels of physical activity and the distribution of subcutaneous fat. Storing your weight around your waist or midriff is known as abdominal obesity and this measurement is much more closely correlated to your risk of chronic disease than your BMI value alone. So on this plan the measurement we are specifically going to track is your waist circumference.

Body Measurements

Before you start my 28-day Step Counter Diet you will need to take the following measurements:

Your weight
Your waist measurement
Your navel measurement (this is the measurement around the midriff, level with your belly button)

You will need to record these measurements on days 1, 7, 14, 21 and 28, the last day of the plan. You can note them down here to see at a glance how much you've achieved (or lost, I should say!)

	WEIGHT	WAIST	NAVEL
Day 1			
Day 7			
Day 14			
Day 21			
Day 28			
Finish Line			

You may also want to take additional body measurements, such as your chest, hips and thighs, so you can track your progress. Many of my clients have found this very motivating, as you will definitely see your body change shape elsewhere too! I suggest you only record these measurements on Day 1 and Day 28, the last day of the plan. It is likely that the changes you experience will be slightly slower for these body parts, although your clothes will most definitely feel more comfortable as you progress through the plan.

	CHEST	HIPS	THIGHS
Day 1			
Day 28			
Finish Line			

Over the 28 days I will ask you to record your weight and waist measurements on the Preview and Review charts at the beginning and end of every week. (These are in the charts section on page 75.) If you have a tendency to weigh yourself every day I'd strongly urge you not to do this when following my plan, and weigh yourself at the end of each week instead. Daily weight changes tend not to reflect real changes in body shape and are more reflective of shifts in fluid retention. This means your weight may appear to go up on some days, which (depending on what you have been doing!) may not be a true reflection of your progress.

Fitness Measurements

Just as you record how your body measurements change, I'd also like you to record how your fitness improves. This can be done very simply, by walking a set distance as fast as you can and recording the time it takes you to cover the distance as well as your heart rate before and after. You will need to do this test at the very start of the plan and also on day 28. Please do this – you will be so surprised by how much your body can improve in just 28 days.

On my 28-day programme we walk as fast as we can for one kilometre. If you are a complete novice to walking and exercise I suggest you complete a timed walk for ½ km. If you don't have a set distance of 1 km, don't worry. Just find your own timed route, ideally one as flat as possible. The route I use on the course is actually beside a park. One length of the park is 250 metres so we walk the length of the park 4 times to complete 1 km as fast as we can.

Before you start your timed walk, record your heart rate for 1 minute. This can be taken at your wrist or your neck. See Box on page 11 for information on how to take this. Immediately after completing the walk you need to take your heart rate for 1 minute then once again after 1 minute of recovery. Record your heart rate results and the time it took you to walk on the chart below. If you are out and about and don't want to carry your book everywhere, just grab a piece of paper and a pencil to jot your results down, then fill in the chart when you get back home.

You should walk the distance *as fast as possible* to get a true indication of your fitness. And remember you need to record your heart rate three times: before the walk, straight after the walk, and then again after a 1-minute recovery time.

	DATE	TIME TO COMPLETE	HR ON COMPLETION	HR AFTER 1 MINUTE
START Day 1				
END Day 28				

The Charts

To guide you through the 28 days I have provided a number of handy charts. There are 28 Day Charts for each day of the plan and 4 Preview and Review charts for each week.

THE DAY CHARTS

You need to fill in these charts every day. There is one for each of the 28 days on the plan. The day charts are so easy to follow – and they allow you to track your road to success!

Remember you can also print off these charts from my web site: www.joannahall.com

TAKING YOUR HEART RATE

You can take your pulse either at your wrist (radial pulse) or at the side of your neck (carotid pulse). You can feel your radial pulse by tracing a line down from the base of your thumb. Place the tips of your index and middle fingers (not the thumb, which has a pulse of its own) over the artery and apply light pressure.

Some people find it hard to locate their radial pulse. In particular, your pulse after exercise is easier to find at the carotid, which is to the side of the larynx. Do not apply heavy pressure to the carotid artery, because it contains baroreceptors which sense increases in pressure and can consequently slow the heart rate.

Another very accurate and easy way to measure your heart rate is with a portable heart rate monitor. There are a number of these on the market, and they consist of a chest strap containing electrodes that pick up the electrical activity of your heart. They are generally a lot more accurate than taking the pulse manually as they pick up your actual heart rate as opposed to your pulse rate.

The most important requirement is to *record accurately*. I know filling in the charts may seem a chore but it really will make you focus on the plan more.

PREVIEW AND REVIEW CHARTS

On days 1, 7, 14, 21 and 28 you need to complete your Preview and Review charts.

Preview Charts

The Preview Charts help you plan your week ahead, encouraging you to decide when you will have time for your exercises and to address any difficulties you feel might hinder your efforts in the next 7 days. Previewing is vitally important.

Filling in the Preview Charts

Read the goals for this week, depending on whether you are a *Walking Whiz* or a *Walking Novice*

- Tick the days you will be able to complete your walking exercise and state your targets (in number of steps and number of minutes)
- Tick the days you will be able to complete your abdominal exercises
- List your weekly challenges
- Tick the category you think your week will fall into: Progressive, Maintenance or Damage Limitation

Next tick the category you think will best apply to the week ahead: **progressive**, **maintenance** or **damage limitation**.

A **Progressive** week is one where you feel 95% confident you can complete all the aspects of the plan you have committed to on your Preview chart. You feel good about yourself, you feel motivated by planning ahead, and feel happy that you can deal with any little blips that may come your way.

A **Maintenance** week is one where you feel 75% confident that you can complete your programme goals for the next 7 days. You feel you may not be able to do all the daily walking goals and you may have a few things to deal with that could make following the plan hard but you feel you can give it your best shot. You feel confident that these little blips are not going to be a real hindrance to your efforts.

A **Damage Limitation** week is one where you feel your life is not conducive to following the plan – perhaps the children are breaking up from school, the washing machine has flooded the floor, it's your time of the month, you have major hassles at work and you have guests all weekend. This kind of week happens. You need to acknowledge that, but don't think "I'll drop the plan this week, have a complete rest and pick it up again next week"! Limit the damage and pick one thing on the plan you can do all week. Perhaps it is your tummy exercises or perhaps it is completing half the daily walking goals instead of all of them. Think carefully and plan – you can Limit the Damage, and limiting the damage is all part of building your template of success.

The first step to limiting the damage is *acknowledging* it is going to be a Damage Limitation week on your Preview Chart.

Review Charts

The Review Charts allow you to look back over the past 7 days and see how you did. They let you give yourself a pat on the back for your progress but also let you assess whether what you are expecting from yourself is realistic. The Review charts act as a reality check – keeping you on track and helping to build a template of success.

Filling in the Review Charts

- Tick the days you completed your daily walking exercise and state the *actual* number of steps and minutes walked
- Tick the days you completed your abdominal exercises
- Tick the category that you feel your week actually fell in to: Progressive, Maintenance or Damage Limitation

The principles

The Energy Gap

If you want to lose weight you have to create an Energy Gap – put simply you have to create as big a gap as possible between the number of calories you consume through food and drink and the number of calories you expend through moving your body. The amount of calories you consume through food and drink needs to decrease while the amount of calories you expend through moving your body has to increase. The bigger the energy gap you create on a consistent basis the greater your success will be. The Step Counter Diet will help you create an Energy Gap, using easily implemented exercise and eating principles to help you lose weight and inches while still enjoying your food. At the end of the 28 days your body will burn more calories – even when you're asleep!

The Eating Principles

There are a number of eating principles that make the plan successful. The plan is designed around these principles, and knowing the logic and science behind them will help you understand how and why my plan is successful.

PRINCIPLE NUMBER ONE : CARB CURFEW

This is your Golden Rule

Carb Curfew means no bread, pasta, rice potatoes or cereal after 5pm for your evening meal. You can eat them for your breakfast, lunch and snacks but you can't eat them after 5pm. You just say no at this time!

Putting Carb Curfew into practice will also help you get a better balance of nutrients. Not only will you get more essential vitamins and minerals from fruit and vegetables in your evening meal, helping you to hit the recommended 5 portions of fruit and veg a day, but you will be optimising your nutrition without having to work too hard.

PRINCIPLE NUMBER 2: FRONTLOAD YOUR DAY

Frontloading your day is about eating your food when your body needs it. Don't skip breakfast – the most important meal of the day – and if you don't have time for a decent lunch try eating it in two halves. If you do this you will be supplying your body with energy at the most critical time – during the day when you are at your most active.

Carb Curfew and frontloading your day work together so that you wake up hungry ready for your breakfast. If you have stuffed your face the night before, you will wake up with a "food hangover" and not be able to enjoy your breakfast – and then the whole cycle begins again, creating a bottom heavy weight gain day rather than a frontloaded weight managing day.

A weight gain day:

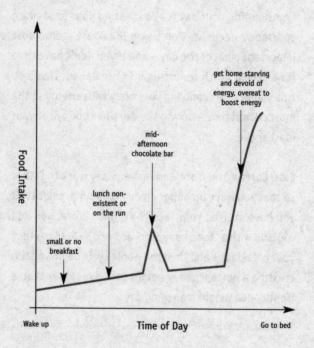

Net effect:

Total calories high. Calories highest when body calorie needs lowest.

A weight managing day:

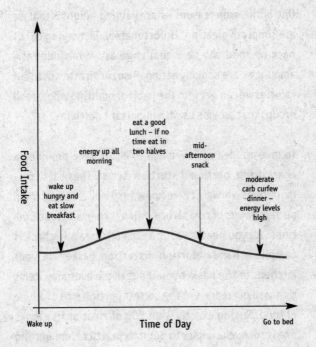

Net effect:

Total calories level but energy levels high all day – improving concentration and enabling you to do structured exercise.

PRINCIPLE NUMBER 3: STOP PORTION DISTORTION

One of the main reasons we are gaining weight is that we are simply overeating. Unfortunately, just trying to cut back on food can be a challenge as we misjudge the amount we are actually eating. Also, in an attempt to cut calories we can get into the habit of omitting whole food groups that provide us with important nutrients.

To give an idea of how much to eat, I have provided a chart using 'portion distortion items'. These are common items whose size we know very well, making them perfect points of comparison when it comes to food portions. All you need to do to keep your meals in check is compile a handy 'portion distortion basket' in your kitchen. In the basket you'll put these everyday items that visually represent the correct portion size of a type of food. Seeing exactly what 80g of meat or fish looks like is so much simpler to put into practice than getting your scales out each time. For example, the amount of meat in a single portion should be no larger than a deck of cards.

FOOD TYPES ITEM	PORTION DISTORTION ITEM	WHAT IT DOES TO YOUR BODY
Nuts and cheese	Golfball	Gives very dense source of energy
Meat and fish	Deck of cards	Builds muscle important for burning calories and healing
Oils and fats	One die	Densest source of energy your body can consume
Vegetables	Tennis ball	Vitamins, minerals and anti oxidants
Starchy carbs	Computer mouse	Fuels muscles for daily activity

PRINCIPLE NUMBER 4: GET YOUR CALCIUM

There is a growing body of evidence that calcium can play a crucial role in our attempts to achieve healthy weight loss. Although the specific scientific mechanisms are not as yet fully understood it is thought that individuals who have low calcium intakes have an increased ability to store excess calories as body fat. Conversely, high levels of dietary calcium can increase your body's ability to burn off fat.

PRINCIPLE NUMBER 5: ENJOY THE RIGHT CARBS!

When it comes to giving you energy, carbs such as grains, fruits and vegetables are the hands down winner. The popularity of low carb diets has given carbs a bad name, but there is no refuting the scientific consensus. Your muscles are fuelled with glycogen, which is a form of the carbohydrate glucose – another name for sugar. This means that carbs are the most expedient source of energy, because they can be used directly to power your muscles without having to be converted first. In addition, your body needs carbs to burn fat when you exercise – so cutting out carbs entirely is not a good idea and getting the right carbs is important for your energy levels and your health.

Consuming foods with a low glycemic index (GI) value is thought to give you a slower release of glucose into your blood stream – helping to keep your blood sugar levels more stable and minimise cravings. Some experts believe that eating low GI foods may help the body burn fat more efficiently.

The **glycemic index** (GI) is a ranking system for carbohydrates based on their effect on blood glucose levels over time. Carbohydrates that break down quickly during digestion, and so have a rapid effect on blood glucose levels, have the highest glycemic indices. Carbohydrates that break down slowly, releasing glucose gradually into the blood stream, have low glycemic indices.

LOW GI 50 OR UNDER	MODERATE GI 50–70	HIGH GI 70 AND OVER
Yoghurt	Brown rice	White rice
Lentils	Banana	Cornflakes
Apples	Sweetcorn	White bread
Kelloggs All-Bran	Cous Cous	Shredded wheat
		Weetabix
Pumpernickel bread		
Porridge	Honey	Bagel
Butter beans	Sweet potato	Parsnips, carrots
Kidney beans		Baked potato
Chick peas	Stoneground wholewheat bread	Sports drinks
Milk	Oatcakes	French Fries
Dried apricots	Raisins	Watermelon

PRINCIPLE NUMBER 6: PICK THE RIGHT PROTEIN

Although many nutritionists are still wary about the potential dangers of high protein diets, consuming slightly more protein than you normally do can be an effective tool for weight loss as it helps you stay fuller for longer. The Step Counter Diet is NOT a low carb plan, but is instead based on a slightly higher intake of protein and a moderate intake of carbohydrate.

Eating protein, particularly after exercise, can also help stimulate muscle building and this has a direct effect on improving your body's ability to burn more fat.

Finally: limit your fats (especially unhealthy saturated ones) and sugar alcohols!

Now it's time to put these eating principles into practice. To help you do this, I have included some recipe suggestions in the recipe section at the end (see page 187).

The Exercise Principles

Exercise is an important part of the Step Counter Diet and is essential to creating that Energy Gap! (See page 17) But before you start panicking about how hard you have to work – relax. The exercise in the plan is simple: it is based on walking and just five tummy exercises. So all you need is a pair of good comfortable walking shoes and enough space to get on the floor for your tummy exercises. You get to choose which walking and tummy programme is right for you and that's it – simple!

Just as there are a number of principles behind the eating programme so there are a number of principles behind the exercise plan. Knowing the reasons for these principles will help you to understand the things I ask you to do.

Have faith in the programme and learn why it will give you such great results!

PRINCIPLE NUMBER 1: MOVE MORE, MORE OFTEN

If you have read any of my books and followed any of my programmes before, you will be familiar with the concept of Navigating the 24! Navigating the 24 is all about not trying to bust a gut every time you do exercise but more about increasing your overall activity levels right through each and every day. Encouraging you to "move more, more often", whether at work or in your leisure time.

All these extra times when you can be more physically active do add up. Think of it this way: there are 24 hours in the day and 7 days in the week. That makes 168 hours in each week. Let's say we have the luxury of getting 10 hours of sleep each night (10 just keeps the arithmetic simple). This leaves us 98 hours (168 - 70 = 98 hours) when we are awake and able to be physically active. Let's suppose we do exercise three times a week for an hour each time, as this is the amount we are generally advised to take and the maximum most people feel they can squeeze into a busy life. This still leaves us with 95 hours (98 - 3 = 95 hours) when we can physically move our bodies.

So what I am asking you to do is give me a little bit more physical activity right through your day. Have a look at the table below and you will soon see that "moving more, more often" can actually be the foundation stone of your physical fitness and weight loss approach.

WHY GYM VISITS ARE NO SUBSTITUTE FOR AN ACTIVE LIFESTYLE

Less active person	kcals
Get someone else to iron while you sit down	34
Get someone else to Hoover while you sit down	11
Prepare pre-sliced vegetables	3
Microwave a ready meal	3
Drive children half-mile to school	11
Drive three miles to work	24
Use lift to travel up four floors	1
Chat with colleagues for 20mins at lunchtime	26
Shop by internet	17
Watch TV for two hours	175
Mow lawn with power mower for 10 mins	50
Read newspaper for half an hour	34
Basic Total	**389**
Compensatory gym workout (60 mins)	403
REVISED TOTAL	**792**

On a representative day, the less active person uses 30% of the calories of the active person. If the less active person compensates by going to the gym he or she still uses 40% less calories than the active person who does not use the gym.

Active person	kcals	Difference
Iron for 30 minutes	77	43
Vacuum for 10 minutes	40	29
Wash, slice & chop veg	28	25
Cook for 30 minutes	67	64
Walk children half-mile to school	56	45
Cycle three miles to work	135	111
Climb four flights of stairs	11	10
Walk and chat for 20 mins	78	52
Walk 1 mile to shop and back	311	294
Take a brisk one-hour walk	336	161
Mow lawn using hand mower	68	18
Play with children for ½ hour	94	60
	1301	912
No gym workout	0	-403
TOTAL	1301	

Energy costs are for a 10st (63.5kg) person. Source: British Heart Foundation health promotion unit, University of Oxford.

One benefit of moving more and more often is that you don't necessarily need to change your kit each time you take your structured exercise – you just need a comfortable pair of walking shoes.

The double bonus

Because you will be a lot more physically active your calorie burn will benefit in two ways – you burn a few extra calories every time you move and you keep your metabolism revved up right through the day. In reality this means you burn an extra 2 calories a minute. That may not sound like much, but add it up over 24 hours, 7 days a week, 4 weeks every month, 12 months a year and you soon notch up an extra 1 million calories a year!

PRINCIPLE NUMBER TWO: TAKE STRUCTURED EXERCISE

This is when you put on your walking shoes and complete your daily walking goals. Taking structured exercise works in conjunction with "moving more, more often", so even though my plan encourages you to be much more physically active throughout the day, taking time out to exercise is still important.

Firstly, it is your opportunity to improve your fitness. Moving more throughout the day will contribute to your overall calorie expenditure but to impact your fitness and to maximise your calorie burn the intensity of your exercise is also important. Following the daily walking tips and weekly walking goals will automatically make you increase your walking intensity – so I've already taken care of that for you.

Secondly, your structured exercise is not purely about achieving a calorie burn. This may be an initial motivation to get you moving but as you progress through the 28-day plan you will soon feel many other benefits – your energy will improve, you'll sleep better and you'll feel great! Feeling better about yourself is such an important aspect of the plan and I cannot express what a wonderful motivator it is.

Every day you need to set aside some time for your structured exercise walks. Walking is the simplest, easiest and cheapest exercise you can do. Whether you are already an experienced walker, pounding that pavement regularly, or you are more familiar with the sofa, the 28-day walking plan is suited to all. And what's more, it delivers results. It will get you out of the door, moving your body and cranking up your calorie burn. And working alongside my Step Counter Diet plan it will help you melt away fat and inches.

Why this works

Evidence from the National Registry of Weight Loss in the US has shown that changing your eating behaviour and getting 150 minutes or more of moderate-intensity physical activity a week will give good long term weight loss.

Getting 200 minutes of moderate-intensity physical activity will give even better long term weight loss.

PRINCIPLE NUMBER 3: COMMIT TO DOING YOUR TUMMY EXERCISES

Together, the abdominals form one of the few muscle groups in your body that can be trained each day. The flat, firm, strong abdominals provide stability for the whole of your body so training them everyday is beneficial to your posture and your body shape. If you can't commit to doing them every day, don't worry, because as long as you are doing them at least three times a week you will see the inches come off. They are so quick to do – all you need is just 7 minutes to whiz through the tummy exercises.

SECTION 2

the plan
in practice

What you have
to do

Follow the quiz below to find out if you are a Walking Novice or a Walking Whiz.

Complete your daily walking goals in your structured exercise sessions. These are your timed structured walks and the targets can be found in the Weekly Previews (see charts section page 75).

Increase your overall levels of physical activity with your lifestyle exercise and occupation exercise. These are the step targets you need to achieve each day in addition to the ones you achieve through your structured exercise.

Choose the Right Walking Level for You

First you need to decide the level that best describes
you – are you a Walking Novice or a Walking Whiz?

Fill in the quiz below to find out if you are a Walking
Novice or a Walking Whiz – this is based on your walking fitness as well as the amount of walking you may
already achieve with your occupation or lifestyle activity. This is just a guideline to help direct you to the
most appropriate walking programme for you.

Do you take 3 hours or more a week of
cardiovascular exercise – of an intensity
sufficient to make you sweat?   **(yes/no)**

Does your job involve regular physical activity –
getting up and moving around at least once an
hour?   **(yes/no)**

Do you regularly walk when taking care of errands?   **(yes/no)**

Do you enjoy active leisure pursuits
(participating in sport or games) in addition
to more sedentary ones (watching TV, reading
or fishing)?   **(yes/no)**

If you answered mostly 'yes', you are a Walking Whiz. If you answered mostly 'no', you are a Walking Novice. But all that will change!

Complete the Daily Exercise Goals

Now that you have found out whether you are a Walking Whiz or a Walking Novice you can choose between the two programmes on the Weekly Previews (page 75). For example, the walking goal for a Novice in the first week is 15 minutes continuous walking plus 5000 steps on the pedometer per day, while the goal for a Whiz is 30 minutes continuous walking plus 7000 steps on the pedometer.

Why this Amount of Exercise?

I want you to feel confident that your efforts will be rewarded, and I believe it is important for you to understand why I am asking you to do this. Obviously your motivation will fluctuate over the 28 days but understanding the logic behind what I am asking you to do is important to helping you stay on track.

Walking at a brisk pace will give you a calorie burn of approximately 5 calories a minute. Research has shown that burning 2800 calories a week through physical activity will, in conjunction with a sensible eating plan, result in weight and inch loss. I've taken all the planning out of it so all you need to do is follow and commit to my plan. You *can* do this – let's get a grip and go for it!

The available evidence suggests that we should all be walking a minimum of 150 minutes a week, just to stay healthy. The Chief Medical Officer recommends we break this down to walking for 30 minutes five times a week. For weight loss, taking at least 280 minutes of exercise a week has been shown to be effective. Individuals who have already lost weight and wish to keep it off need to walk for more than 200 minutes a week to avoid weight regain. Walking at a brisker pace will improve your cardiovascular fitness as well as increasing your overall calorie expenditure. You can follow the daily walking tips as well as the weekly walking goals to increase your walking intensity while having fun at the same time.

The pedometer

The pedometer is just about the best little fitness tool you can have – it is your daily reminder of how active you are.

It is also a great tool to accompany your walking plan, allowing you to record the number of steps you take a day. Your pedometer works by measuring the up-and-down motion of your hip as you walk. It will also measure other movements you perform, like walking up and down stairs or getting in and out of your car. But don't worry about this distorting your daily total – activity can be accumulated from other forms of movement in addition to walking.

You should clip your pedometer onto your belt directly above your knee. As with any piece of equipment there can be an element of error so use the pedometer as a guide as well as your reference tool. But as long as you wear your pedometer correctly, you should find it will measure the number of steps you take with great accuracy.

At the end of each day, take off your pedometer and write down the number of steps you take on your day chart. You should be aiming for at least 10,000 steps a day in order to prevent weight gain and maximise your health.

If you ever find yourself without your pedometer, you can follow this guide to measure your steps:

30 minutes moderately paced walking is equivalent to approximately 4000 steps

45 minutes moderately paced walking is equivalent to approximately 7500 steps

60 minutes briskly paced walking is equivalent to approximately 10,000 steps

WHAT IS THE SIGNIFICANCE OF 10,000 STEPS?

There is evidence that walking 10,000 steps a day can lead to significant health benefits. If done daily it can make you feel better and can help reduce the risk of developing serious illnesses such as heart disease, some cancers, diabetes and depression. Put another way, the 10,000 steps message is merely encouraging you not to sit down for too long. If you get up and move every 30 minutes, you'll soon clock up those steps. In addition, getting into the habit of taking 10,000 steps a day becomes the foundation for your physical activity and exercise. When life gets busy the first thing that tends to be put to one side is structured exercise. When this happens, accumulating your 10,000 steps a day through your daily life will still contribute to your overall calorie burn. Studies have shown that taking 10,000 steps a day without any adjustment to your diet will maintain your weight.

How to Wear Your Pedometer

1 Slide the clip onto your belt or waistband. The most common placement is directly above and in line with your knee. However, you may have to experiment to find the best placement for your body type. If your tummy protrudes over your waistband or belt, it may cause the pedometer to tilt and not work properly. If this is the case try wearing the pedometer more to the side of your body. **Take care to position the pedometer in such a way that you are not likely to hit the reset button accidentally when it is in use.**

2 If your pedometer comes with a security strap, attach the strap's clip onto a belt loop, waistband or belt. You will find more information about your free pedometer on page 212.

Frequently asked questions

I have heard that I should be active for 30 minutes a day, for 5 or more days a week. Where does this message fit in with the 10,000 steps programme?

This advice is still valid. Walking briskly for 30 minutes a day has been proven to reduce the risk of disease in many areas. It is the current guideline given by most UK and US health organisations. It has also been shown that the 30 minutes can be split into two lots of 15 minutes, or three lots of 10 minutes, and still bring significant health benefits.

Getting started with a physical activity routine is a major step on the way to a physically active lifestyle. Unfortunately we cannot bottle the benefits from our current exercise habits for use at some point in the future. Physical activity has to be sustained over the long term to accrue the significant health benefits that are associated with it. Even former athletes who quit exercise altogether at the end of their careers have similar rates of chronic disease as people who've never exercised. Finding a physical activity routine that you can sustain throughout your lifespan is critical for deriving maximum benefit. Importantly, it's never too late to start. People who take up exercise in their 60s can still achieve significant health benefits

Will I lose weight just by doing the walking programme?

The daily walking target of 10,000 steps is widely recognised as the daily target to aim for in order to see improvements in your health and weight management. But while taking 10,000 steps a day can improve your fitness, without any dietary changes it will not be enough for you to see weight loss. If your primary aim is to lose weight you will need to follow the eating principles as well as the walking targets. However, if you feel you may find it difficult to cope with both the walking and the diet, then just follow the walking plan. You will definitely feel better, see improvements in your body shape and find that your clothes fit better. Some of my clients who have completed a 28-day programme focusing on the walking alone have experienced such improvements in their self-esteem, confidence and energy levels that they have immediately enrolled in another 28-day plan and addressed their eating as well.

Taking 10,000–12,000 steps a day and changing your eating habits will result in weight loss and inch loss. If you want to experience weight loss but are not prepared to adjust your eating habits, studies have shown you will need to take in the region of 20,000 steps a day. Even without weight loss regular moderate exercise will reduce your abdominal fat and insulin resistance. This improved fitness is important for decreasing risk of chronic diseases. So even if you do not decrease your total weight by following my 28-day walking programme you will alter your abdominal fat and get great health outcomes.

Step trade offs

If you really can't resist the odd snack, then Step Trade Offs are the answer. Step Trade Offs are intended to give you a guide to the number of steps you will need to take in order to burn off those calories. **Please bear in mind that this is a guideline only, as portion sizes, calorie content and walking speed are all variable.**

I have provided tables for all major food groups in the Trade Off section on pages 153–208, which simply list foods, the number of calories they contain, and the number of steps those calories are equivalent to.

The idea is simple: applying the Trade Off means you don't have to deprive yourself of your favourite foods. If you fancy a packet of crisps, go ahead and have them. All you have to do is accumulate the additional steps to the equivalent calorie value. Remember: counting steps to keep your energy gap in the right direction is a tool and not an obsession.

It is worth remembering that:

6 chocolate cookies

OR

One McDonald's Cheeseburger

OR

3 large oranges

= a 3 mile brisk walk or 6000 steps on your pedometer. All of which are equivalent to 300 calories.

You can see that steps can be used to directly cancel out a snack. Any little bit of additional physical activity goes towards justifying that snack and keeping you in energy balance.

So follow the Step Trade Off chart (*see* page 52) to see how you can still enjoy some of the snacks you may be tempted to splurge on. I have also provided figures for some popular junk foods, which you will find here – you may be surprised at the number of steps you will need to burn off that snack indulgence! Remember this is not about saying you can never have snacks or enjoy your food. But this simple Trade Off can quickly and easily put things in perspective as well as encouraging you to increase your overall physical activity levels.

INDULGENCE	CALS	STEPS
1 Chocolate Cookie	86	2150
1 Bagel (standard size)	230	5750
5 cms long Garlic Ciabatta Bread	200	5000
1 Plain Naan Bread	294	7350
1 Chocolate Brownie Cake	328	8200
2 Chocolate Cookies	174	4350
1 Pecan Danish Pastry	287	7175
1 Jam Doughnut	324	8100
1 Shop-bought Blueberry Muffin	438	10950
1 Pain au Chocolat	235	5875
1 McDonald's Big Breakfast	591	14775
1 KFC Fillet Towermeal Burger	656	16400
1 Burger King Whopper with Mayo	678	16950
8 Pizza Express mini Dough Balls	200	5000
1 McDonald's McFlurry Crème Egg	390	9750
1 Pizza Express American Hot Pizza	788	19700
1 Pizza Hut Margherita Stuffed Crust Original	330	8250
1 McDonald's Hot Fudge Sundae	352	8800
1 Fish & Chips	849	21225

INDULGENCE	CALS	STEPS
1 Sushi Fish Box (1 person)	423	10575
2 Thick Pork & Beef Sausages	330	8250
1 Individual Quiche Lorraine	262	6550
1 Tuna Melt sandwich	621	15525
1 ready-made Cheese Sandwich	618	15450
1 large can Heinz Baked Beans	303	7575
1 ready-meal Sweet & Sour Chicken with Rice	440	11000
1 ready-meal Ham & Mushroom Tagliatelle	486	12150
1 shop-bought Tuna & Sweetcorn Jacket Potato	333	8325
1 Cheese & Bacon Potato Skins	241	6025
1 McDonald's Chocolate Milk Shake	403	10075
1 Burger King King Size Salted French Fries	539	13475
1 can Fanta Lemon Drink	165	4125
1 Blockbuster carton Salted Popcorn	121	3025
3 Roast Potatoes	280	7000

Walking troubleshooting

Walking Technique

Walking is the simplest form of exercise you can take – you just put one foot in front of another! But there are a few tweaks to your walking technique that can help you get more out of your walking, burn more calories, minimise your risk of aches and pains and just make the whole experience a lot more enjoyable.

KEEP YOUR HEAD UP

Keep your eye line looking ahead as you walk, so you avoid always looking down on the floor in front of you. This decreases neck strain and improves posture – you want to see improvements in the future so keep looking ahead and stop looking down! In bright light or drizzling rain it is common to tilt your head down to avoid the glare or the wet. To improve your walking posture, wear a hat or sunglasses so you can keep you chin up and parallel to the ground.

ROCK AND ROLL

For a more efficient, less jarring stride, visualise your feet as rockers on a rocking chair. Start each step on the heel and rock your foot forward until you roll onto your toes. Pick up your speed so you're rolling the foot with each stride.

WARM UP SLOWLY

Five minutes of easy walking can help you log more miles by warming up your muscles before a workout. Wrap up with 5 minutes of easy walking and you'll finish with a more enjoyable impression of your workout, making you less likely to skip it tomorrow.

Tips to Avoid Aches and Pains

As you start your walking programme you may come across a few little niggles in your body. This is quite normal and to be expected if you are new to exercise. However, to keep you walking stronger and longer and burning more energy try these little tips to avoid common problems:

AVOID SHIN PAIN – THE FOOT ROLL

Standing with your feet almost together roll up onto your toes, hold for 2 seconds and roll back down. Then roll onto the outside of your feet, hold both for 2 seconds and roll back down. Next roll onto your heels with the toes off the ground, hold for 2 seconds and roll back down. Do this sequence 10 times before every walk.

AVOID KNEE PAIN – THE STRAIGHT LEG RAISE

Sit on the ground with your leg extended in front of you, right leg bent and right foot flat on the ground. Place your hands behind you and sit up straight. With your left foot flexed, contract your left thigh and raise your leg 6–12 inches off the floor. Hold for 5 seconds and then lower. Do 10 lifts, and then switch sides. Perform the sequence 2–4 times a week.

AVOID LEG ACHES – THE HIP AND CALF STRETCH

Standing with your feet together, step your right foot in front of you about 3–4 feet so both feet are pointing forward. Bend your right knee so it is just above but not in front of your right foot. Check both big toes are facing forward. Keep your left leg straight and your left heel on the ground to feel a stretch in your left calf. Flatten your lower back and tuck your pelvis so that you also feel a stretch in the front of your hip. Hold for 4–7 slow deep breaths, release and repeat on the other side. Stretch each leg two times after each walk.

AVOID SORE CALVES – THE CALF STRETCH

Stand close to a tree or lamppost and place the ball of your foot on the post or trunk so the heel is still on the ground but the ball of the foot is resting up on the post. Bend the knee towards the post; you should feel the stretch in the lower part of the calf. Hold for 10–15 seconds and repeat twice on each side. Do this at the end of each walk.

AVOID UPPER ARM TENSION – THE UPPER BODY STRETCH

Stand with your feet about shoulder-distance apart and raise your right arm over your head, bending your elbow so your right hand is behind your head. Place your left hand on your right elbow and gently pull your elbow to the left, allowing your upper body to bend slightly to the left. Hold for 4–7 deep breaths, release and repeat on the other side. Stretch each side two times after every walk.

The abdominal exercises

Choosing the Right Tummy Exercises for You

First, decide which level of tummy exercises is best for you. Choosing the right exercises is important: opting for harder ones than you are ready for can mean you don't perform the exercises correctly and don't get a flat tummy. Harder in this case *does not mean you are going to get better results*.

Choose the No Neck Pain Programme if you:

- Are new to abdominal exercises
- Suffer from neck pain with your abdominal exercises
- Have a popped out belly
- Just had a baby

If you tend to do a lot of abdominal work but feel frustrated with never getting the results you want, I'd suggest you follow the No Neck Pain programme for the first week to help you really master the techniques and then move on to the advanced programme from day 8 onwards.

Choose the Advanced Programme if you:

- Are familiar with abdominal exercises
- Have mastered the rib-hip connection (see opposite)
- Suffer from no back or neck pain.

Once you have chosen which level suits you, simply follow the respective programme, incorporating the exercises described into your daily goals. You should also plan when you'll be able to do the abdominal exercises using your weekly Preview Charts (page 75).

THE RIB-HIP CONNECTION

Before you start any abdominal exercises, make sure you have a connection between your ribs and your hips. This will help you contract the abdominals before you lift and ensure you are in the correct anatomical position for your spine.

Here is what you do: when lying on the floor, place your thumb on your bottom ribs and your fingers at the top of the hip bone, then draw these two points together with a small contraction of the abdominal muscles. Your spine should be in a neutral position. This neutral position will vary from person to person depending on the shape of the spine. However, there should be a small space between the floor and your back. Keep the rib-hip connection to establish trunk stability.

Once you have mastered this technique, you will really start to see an improvement in your abdominal training.

No Neck Pain Flat Tummy Programme

HEEL SLIDES

Start position: lie on your back with your arms by your sides, legs stretched out in front of you. Bend one knee, so the foot is flat on the floor by the knee of the straight leg. Keeping your hips still, pull in your tummy muscles and slowly draw the heel in towards the other foot. Keep the foot relaxed and slowly extend the leg out along the floor again. Do 8 of these on each side.

BELT PULLS

Start position: first put on a snugly fitting belt. Buckle it so it fits snugly around your waist. Get onto all fours with your hands under your wrists and your knees under your hips. Start with your abdominals relaxed – you may find your tummy is touching your belt. Now, keeping the back straight, firmly draw the abdominal muscles so you "create" space between your tummy and your belt. You should be able to slip your fingers in between your belt and your tummy. Hold this position for 30 seconds, breathing smoothly throughout. Relax for 10 seconds and repeat 5 times.

BELT PULL BALANCE

Start position: on all fours with your snug fitting belt as above. Keep your back straight as you extend opposite arm and leg. Now draw in your abdominal muscles firmly to create the space between your belt and your tummy. This is more challenging so start off holding for 10 seconds and build up to 5 sets of 30 second holds.

DEAD BUG

Start position: lie on your back and lift your legs off the floor, so your knees are over your hips and your arms are directly over your shoulders. Hold this position for 20 seconds, keeping as still as possible and firmly pulling your abdominals into the base of your spine. Relax down for 10 seconds and repeat 5 times.

BREASTBONE LIFT

Start position: lie on the floor face up, knees slightly bent and feet on the floor – but far enough away from your bottom so you feel as if your toes are just about to come off the floor. Place your hands at the side of your head and lift your head off the floor. From here lift no more than 2 inches / 10 centimetres from the breastbone. Hold this small lift for 4 counts then lower back to the start position and lower the head to the floor. Repeat 8 times.

Advanced Flat Tummy Programme

MOVING DEAD BUG

Start position: adopt the dead bug position, hands directly over shoulders and knees slightly extended to engage your abdominals. Slowly lower the same leg and arm towards the floor, keeping the same distance between the hand and the knee. Gently "kiss" the floor with your heel and slowly lift the arm and leg back up to the starting dead bug position. Repeat 16 times.

FULL ROLL UP

Start position: lie on the floor, legs extended straight out in front of you and arms directly over your shoulders. Slowly curl up one vertebra at a time using your abdominals and not your legs. Keep the spine curved and reach forward with your hands towards your feet. Sit straight with shoulders directly over hips and slowly curl down one vertebra at a time. Repeat 10–12 times.

AB REACH

Start position: on your back with your knees slightly bent so your feet slightly come off the floor. Lift your head off the floor, leading from your breastbone, and place your hands by your thighs. Lift from the breast bone about 2 inches, trying to reach further around your thighs with your hands if your can. Lower back to your start position and extend your arms above your head, keeping your shoulders off the floor. Do 8–12 of these.

TOWEL OBLIQUE REACH

Start position: take a large towel and roll it into a sausage shape. Lie on your side so your hip is placed on top of the towel. Make sure your hips are stacked up on top of each other and pull in your abdominals tightly to avoid you toppling either forwards or backwards. You may need to play around with the towel position so you can use your waist muscles more as you lift. Extend your bottom arm along the floor and your top arm in front of you. Keeping the waist long, extend out through the top of the head as your lift your body up sideways. You should feel your waist muscles tightening. Slowly lower down. Repeat 12 times on each side.

STRAIGHT LEG LIFT

Start position: this is a variation on the breastbone lift but is more challenging, with only one leg extended. Start with one leg extended. Place your hands at the side of your head and lift the head off the floor. From here lift no more than 2 inches / 10 centimetres from the breastbone. Hold this small lift for 4 counts and lower back to the start position and lower the head to the floor. Do 8 on each side.

5-day countdown

Now we're just about ready to go! You know what you've got to do and also why – so let's get prepared and let the countdown begin.

This section outlines the things you need to do before you start, based on my experience with clients starting the 28-day programme. I have spread the tips out over 5 days but you could just as easily condense them down into three or less if you are in a hurry to get going. However, a little prior preparation does make a big difference in the long run and will help you get better results and a more successful programme. Always remember a little expression I call the 5 Ps: Prior Preparation Prevents Poor Performance!

5 Days to go

CHECK YOUR SHOES!

Put your shoes on the table and check them out for signs of wear and tear. Are the heels more worn down on one side? Your shoes may look in good condition from the top but your soles may tell a different story. And if they *are* worn down, they are not going to give you the support you need. You don't have to fork out a fortune to get good walking shoes – but your fitness and your feet are worth the investment. Check your socks at the same time – wearing them will help avoid blisters. Surprisingly, synthetic fibres are better for whisking away odour and perspiration! Check for signs of uneven wear on the heel or ball of the sock as this can create blisters too.

4 Days to go

DIG OUT YOUR WATERPROOFS

Let's have a reality check: the sun is probably not going to stay shining for you every time you go out and walk. But walking in damp weather can actually be very refreshing and enjoyable if you have the right kit on hand – water proofs and a waterproof hat. Baseball caps can be especially useful as the peak can keep the rain and wind out of your eyes. So dig out your water-proofs or borrow a friend's so that you have them ready when it starts to get a little wet and you don't let the rain become an excuse for not doing your exercise!

TEST YOUR FITNESS

Complete your fitness walking test and record your per-formance. Don't put this off – you will find it so rewarding and it will give you such a sense of achieve-ment when you finish the plan. Trust me!

3 Days to go

PLAN YOUR FOOD SHOPPING

Read through the eating principles and make yourself a list of all foods you need for the first week. Having handy containers, freezer bags and frozen fruit and vegetables can make life a lot simpler. You may also want to buy some second skin blister pads and keep them in the cupboard just in case you get a blister. If you order your shopping online do it today so your delivery is ready to start when you are!

2 Days to go

JOT DOWN YOUR MOTIVES

Come up with five motives, jot them down on a piece of paper and store them in a jar or decorative box. These motives will be there to act as reminders when your motivation fails. Keep them in a prominent place like the bathroom or kitchen so you get a little visual reminder of your 28-day plan every time you go in there. Reading reminders such as "fit into that pair of trousers for wedding reception", "lower my choles-terol and improve my health so I can play with the grandchildren" or "get fit so I can sign up for 5K charity event" may just give you that extra jolt to stop a cop-out!

1 Day to go

CREATE A BACK-UP PLAN

Map out three routes near your home, work place, or child's school, of varying lengths – 10, 20, 30 and 40 minutes. This will give you some options on busy days when it may not be possible to complete your walking goal. You may be short of time but creating a back-up plan will stop that day becoming a cop-out.

Now we are ready to go! **Remember, you will need to take your measurements on day one** (*see* page 6 – Chapter 1, Body Measurements)

BACK-UP ROUTES

MY BACK-UP ROUTES ARE:

For 10 minutes of walking _____

For 20 minutes of walking _____

For 30 minutes of walking _____

For 40 minutes of walking _____

Charts

Weekly Preview

START OF WEEK ONE

Week One Walking Goals

Walking Novice: 15 minutes continuous walking plus 5000 steps on your pedometer every day.

Walking Whiz: 30 minutes continuous walking plus 7000 steps on your pedometer.

I will take structured exercise on these days:

	TARGET STEPS	TARGET MINUTES
M	_____	_____
T	_____	_____
W	_____	_____
T	_____	_____
F	_____	_____
S	_____	_____
S	_____	_____

TOTAL STEPS	TOTAL MINUTES
_____	_____

I will do my abdominal exercises on these days:

M ❏
T ❏
W ❏
T ❏
F ❏
S ❏
S ❏

My measurements:

WEIGHT	WAIST	NAVEL	CHEST	HIPS	THIGH

This week my challenges are:

1. _____
2. _____
3. _____
4. _____

I think the week ahead will fall into the following category (circle the relevant one):

Progressive   **Maintenance**   **Damage Limitation**

(*see* page 13 for an explanation of these categories)

date: ———————————

DAY ONE

DAILY WALKING TIP: **Make a statement**
Email four of your friends and tell them you are commencing your 28-day plan.

Structured Exercise: ❑

(tick here if you have completed your structured exercise today, then fill in the number of steps and minutes you managed. You can compare this with your predictions in this week's Preview Chart!)

	TARGET	ACTUAL
Timed structured walk (mins)		
Steps		

Abdominal Exercise: ☐

(tick here if you completed your abdominal exercises today)

date: ——————————————

DAY TWO

DAILY WALKING TIP: **Speed up your arm swing**
To increase your walking pace – speed up your arm swing. You'll find your legs will naturally speed up and fit into a natural faster stride.

Structured Exercise: ❏

(tick here if you have completed your structured exercise today, then fill in the number of steps and minutes you managed. You can compare this with your predictions in this week's Preview Chart!)

	TARGET	ACTUAL
Timed structured walk (mins)		
Steps		

Abdominal Exercise: ❏

(tick here if you completed your abdominal exercises today)

date: ————————————————

DAY THREE

DAILY WALKING TIP: **Dig out a beautiful route**
People who live near trails or walking paths are far
more physically active than those who don't. If there
are none in your neighbourhood, search out your near-
est National Trust park, country house and gardens,
botanical gardens, or reservoirs, then get over to that
area before your reach day 28 and the finish line!

Structured Exercise: ❑

(tick here if you have completed your structured exercise today, then fill in the number of steps and minutes
you managed. You can compare this with your predictions in this week's Preview Chart!)

	TARGET	ACTUAL
Timed structured walk (mins)		
Steps		

Abdominal Exercise: ❑

(tick here if you completed your abdominal exercises
today)

date: _____

DAY FOUR

DAILY WALKING TIP: **Breathe away stress**
Concentrate on breathing in through your nose and out through your mouth for at least the first few minutes of each walk. Focus on draining air into your belly first, before letting the air expand into your rib cage and chest. Deep full breaths help relieve stress and energise your walk and your day.

Structured Exercise: ❑

(tick here if you have completed your structured exercise today, then fill in the number of steps and minutes you managed. You can compare this with your predictions in this week's Preview Chart!)

	TARGET	ACTUAL
Timed structured walk (mins)		
Steps		

Abdominal Exercise: ☐

(tick here if you completed your abdominal exercises
today)

date: ——————————————

DAY FIVE

DAILY WALKING TIP: **Stop aching shins**
This is a common problem when you try to walk faster. To get these muscles up to speed, walk on your heels for 30 seconds only (feet flexed and toes pointing toward the sky). Repeat three more times during your walk on 2 or 3 days a week.

Structured Exercise: ❑

(tick here if you have completed your structured exercise today, then fill in the number of steps and minutes you managed. You can compare this with your predictions in this week's Preview Chart!)

	TARGET	ACTUAL
Timed structured walk (mins)		
Steps		

Abdominal Exercise: ❑

(tick here if you completed your abdominal exercises
today)

date: _____

DAY SIX

DAILY WALKING TIP: **Visualize full glasses**
To help minimize any shin pain or back pain imagine
you have a cup full of water balanced on each hip as
you walk. Pulling in your tummy muscles and lifting up
out of your hips will not only improve your posture and
reduce back ache, but you'll instantly look better too.

Structured Exercise: ❑

(tick here if you have completed your structured exercise today, then fill in the number of steps and minutes
you managed. You can compare this with your predictions in this week's Preview Chart!)

	TARGET	ACTUAL
Timed structured walk (mins)		
Steps		

Abdominal Exercise: ❑

(tick here if you completed your abdominal exercises today)

date: _____

DAY SEVEN

DAILY WALKING TIP: **Reduce the Impact**
If you have a choice of walking terrain between a concrete pavement or an asphalt road, choose the latter because it is softer. But if the road slants towards the curb reverse the direction you walk every couple of days to avoid injuries resulting from walking on uneven surfaces.

Structured Exercise: ❏

(tick here if you have completed your structured exercise today, then fill in the number of steps and minutes you managed. You can compare this with your predictions in this week's Preview Chart!)

	TARGET	ACTUAL
Timed structured walk (mins)		
Steps		

Abdominal Exercise: ❏

(tick here if you completed your abdominal exercises today)

Weekly Review

END OF WEEK ONE

I took structured exercise on the following days:

	ACTUAL STEPS	ACTUAL MINUTES
M	_____	_____
T	_____	_____
W	_____	_____
T	_____	_____
F	_____	_____
S	_____	_____
S	_____	_____

TOTAL STEPS	TOTAL MINUTES
_____	_____

I did my abdominal exercises on:

M   ☐
T   ☐
W   ☐
T   ☐
F   ☐
S   ☐
S   ☐

My measurements:

WEIGHT	WAIST	NAVEL	CHEST	HIPS	THIGH

On reflection my week fell into the following category
(circle the relevant one):

Progressive   **Maintenance**   -   **Damage
                                               Limitation**

Weekly Preview

START OF WEEK TWO

Week Two Walking Goals

Walking Novice: 20 minutes continuous walking plus 8000 steps on your pedometer every day.

Walking Whiz: 40 minutes continuous walking plus 9000 steps on your pedometer.

I will take structured exercise on these days:

	TARGET STEPS	TARGET MINUTES
M	_____	_____
T	_____	_____
W	_____	_____
T	_____	_____
F	_____	_____
S	_____	_____
S	_____	_____
	TOTAL STEPS	**TOTAL MINUTES**
	_____	_____

I will do my abdominal exercises on these days:

M ☐
T ☐
W ☐
T ☐
F ☐
S ☐
S ☐

My weekly challenges/potential cop outs:

1. _____
2. _____
3. _____
4. _____

I think the week ahead will fall into the following category (circle the relevant one):

Progressive   **Maintenance**   **Damage Limitation**

date: _____

DAY EIGHT

DAILY WALKING TIP: **Breathing**
To avoid snatching your breath, and getting a stitch, focus on your breathing technique. Try to take a breath in every 4 counts or strides and take 4 strides or counts to breathe out.

Structured Exercise: ❏

(tick here if you have completed your structured exercise today, then fill in the number of steps and minutes you managed. You can compare this with your predictions in this week's Preview Chart!)

	TARGET	ACTUAL
Timed structured walk (mins)		
Steps		

Abdominal Exercise: ❑

(tick here if you completed your abdominal exercises today)

date: ———————————————

DAY NINE

DAILY WALKING TIP: **Find a tune**
Why not listen to an up-tempo favourite tune as you
walk today – it can get you walking faster.

Structured Exercise: ❏

(tick here if you have completed your structured exercise today, then fill in the number of steps and minutes
you managed. You can compare this with your predictions in this week's Preview Chart!)

	TARGET	ACTUAL
Timed structured walk (mins)		
Steps		

Abdominal Exercise: ❑

(tick here if you completed your abdominal exercises today)

date: ———————————

DAY TEN

DAILY WALKING TIP: **Wear a belt to get a better bottom**
Believe it or not, wearing a belt will help you get a
better backside. Putting on a snugly fitting belt, and
pulling in your abdominals more so you create a space
between the belt and the belly, helps to flatten your
tummy and stabilises your pelvis. This improves the
toning effects on your bottom with each walking
stride!

Structured Exercise: ❏

(tick here if you have completed your structured exercise today, then fill in the number of steps and minutes
you managed. You can compare this with your predictions in this week's Preview Chart!)

	TARGET	ACTUAL
Timed structured walk (mins)		
Steps		

Abdominal Exercise: ❑

(tick here if you completed your abdominal exercises today)

date: —————————————

DAY ELEVEN

DAILY WALKING TIP: **Get out of a slump**
To stand up straight, bend your left arm behind your
waist and grab your right arm at the elbow. This simple
move pulls your shoulders back and down. Hold for
about 10 seconds and then switch arms. Do 2 or 3
times throughout each walk.

Structured Exercise: ❏

(tick here if you have completed your structured exercise today, then fill in the number of steps and minutes
you managed. You can compare this with your predictions in this week's Preview Chart!)

	TARGET	ACTUAL
Timed structured walk (mins)		
Steps		

Abdominal Exercise: ☐

(tick here if you completed your abdominal exercises today)

date: ——————————————

DAY TWELVE

DAILY WALKING TIP: **Keep your hands free**
You can stash away everything you need in a stylish bum bag – things like keys, money and mobile phone. Keeping your hands free will help your walking technique plus allow you to run some errands as you hit your walking target.

Structured Exercise: ❑

(tick here if you have completed your structured exercise today, then fill in the number of steps and minutes you managed. You can compare this with your predictions in this week's Preview Chart!)

	TARGET	ACTUAL
Timed structured walk (mins)		
Steps		

Abdominal Exercise: ❏

(tick here if you completed your abdominal exercises today)

date: ————————————

DAY THIRTEEN

DAILY WALKING TIP: **Don't use weights**
Don't be fooled into thinking walking while holding handweights will make your work out harder and so help you burn more calories. Studies show that for your body to achieve any additional calorie expenditure from carrying handweights you need to hold a minimum of 3 pounds on each hand. This is actually quite a load and the small additional increase in calorie burn is outweighed by the potential strain at the shoulder joint. Adding inclines and hills is a much more efficient way to burn more calories – see tip on day 17.

Structured Exercise: ❏

(tick here if you have completed your structured exercise today, then fill in the number of steps and minutes you managed. You can compare this with your predictions in this week's Preview Chart!)

	TARGET	ACTUAL
Timed structured walk (mins)		
Steps		

Abdominal Exercise: ❑

(tick here if you completed your abdominal exercises today)

date: _____

DAY FOURTEEN

DAILY WALKING TIP: **Take a half time break**
You're off the hook today: walk only half of the recommended time, but do it at a faster pace than usual.
This is a great way to fit in a full workout when your
schedule is tight. You can burn the same number of
calories whether you walk for 3 mph or 20 minutes at
4 mph.

Structured Exercise: ❑

(tick here if you have completed your structured exercise today, then fill in the number of steps and minutes
you managed. You can compare this with your predictions in this week's Preview Chart!)

	TARGET	ACTUAL
Timed structured walk (mins)		
Steps		

Abdominal Exercise: ❑

(tick here if you completed your abdominal exercises today)

Weekly Review

END OF WEEK TWO

I took structured exercise on the following days:

	ACTUAL STEPS	ACTUAL MINUTES
M	_____	_____
T	_____	_____
W	_____	_____
T	_____	_____
F	_____	_____
S	_____	_____
S	_____	_____
	TOTAL STEPS	**TOTAL MINUTES**
	_____	_____

I did my abdominal exercises on:

M ☐
T ☐
W ☐
T ☐
F ☐
S ☐
S ☐

My measurements:

WEIGHT	WAIST	NAVEL	CHEST	HIPS	THIGH

On reflection my week fell into the following category
(circle the relevant one):

Progressive   **Maintenance**   **Damage
                                             Limitation**

Weekly Preview

START OF WEEK THREE

Week Three Walking Goals

Walking Novice: 25 minutes continuous walking plus 9000 steps on your pedometer.

Walking Whiz: 45 minutes continuous walking or 2 bouts of continuous walking totalling 45 minutes plus 9000 steps on your pedometer.

I will take structured exercise on these days:

	TARGET STEPS	TARGET MINUTES
M	_____	_____
T	_____	_____
W	_____	_____
T	_____	_____
F	_____	_____
S	_____	_____
S	_____	_____

TOTAL STEPS	TOTAL MINUTES
_____	_____

I will do my abdominal exercises on these days:

M ☐
T ☐
W ☐
T ☐
F ☐
S ☐
S ☐

My weekly challenges/potential cop outs:

1. _____
2. _____
3. _____
4. _____

I think the week ahead will fall into the following category (circle the relevant one):

Progressive   **Maintenance**   **Damage Limitation**

date: _____

DAY FIFTEEN

DAILY WALKING TIP: **Play with break point**

You can raise your exercise calorie burn by playing with your break point. In your walks this week, try walking for 15 seconds at your break point pace every three minutes.

To find your breakpoint, walk as fast as you can, remembering that speeding up your arm swing will naturally increase the speed of your leg stride. Make sure you maintain good technique and try to progressively increase your walking pace until you feel you are just about to break into a jog. This is your breakpoint. Walking at this pace will feel slightly uncomfortable and difficult so use it to find your optimum walking pace and to boost your calorie burn on some of your structured walking sessions.

Structured Exercise: ❑

(tick here if you have completed your structured exercise today, then fill in the number of steps and minutes you managed. You can compare this with your predictions in this week's Preview Chart!)

	TARGET	ACTUAL
Timed structured walk (mins)		
Steps		

Abdominal Exercise: ❑

(tick here if you completed your abdominal exercises today)

date: ———————————

DAY SIXTEEN

DAILY WALKING TIP: **Review your fitness test**
Remember your fitness walking test route? Today go
and have a practice walk on it as part of your walk.

Structured Exercise: ❑

(tick here if you have completed your structured exercise today, then fill in the number of steps and minutes
you managed. You can compare this with your predictions in this week's Preview Chart!)

	TARGET	ACTUAL
Timed structured walk (mins)		
Steps		

Abdominal Exercise: ❑

(tick here if you completed your abdominal exercises today)

date: _____

DAY SEVENTEEN

DAILY WALKING TIP: **Raise your incline**
Start climbing – hill walking burns up to 60% more calories than walking at the same pace on level ground and it's great for firming your backside. If you are struggling to find a route with an incline, why not go to your local leisure centre or gym and jump on a treadmill? It is easy to do some hill walking using the incline setting.

Structured Exercise: ❏

(tick here if you have completed your structured exercise today, then fill in the number of steps and minutes you managed. You can compare this with your predictions in this week's Preview Chart!)

	TARGET	ACTUAL
Timed structured walk (mins)		
Steps		

Abdominal Exercise:　　　❑

(tick here if you completed your abdominal exercises today)

date: _____

DAY EIGHTEEN

DAILY WALKING TIP: **Change your walking rhythm**
Changing the rhythm of your walk can boost your energy. Instead of the usual 2 count or 4 count step (left right left right) count in threes. Chant a positive mantra, such as "Yes I can!"

Structured Exercise: ❑

(tick here if you have completed your structured exercise today, then fill in the number of steps and minutes you managed. You can compare this with your predictions in this week's Preview Chart!)

	TARGET	ACTUAL
Timed structured walk (mins)		
Steps		

Abdominal Exercise: ❑

(tick here if you completed your abdominal exercises today)

date: _____

DAY NINETEEN

DAILY WALKING TIP: **Add lunges**

Add 8 lunges after each 10 minutes of walking this week. If you are a Walking Novice – introduce 4 every 5 minutes. Stand in neutral position. Take a large step back with one leg, ensuring the front knee stays over the ankle and is not turned in. The extended leg should have a slight bend at the knee, while the rear heel should be off the ground. Lunge by bending your rear leg so that the knee comes close to the ground, making sure to energize into your back heel to help you use your buttock muscles more effectively. Draw up through your abdominals as you lift your leg back to the start position. Do 4 lunges with each leg (2 if you are a Walking Novice.)

Structured Exercise: ❑

(tick here if you have completed your structured exercise today, then fill in the number of steps and minutes you managed. You can compare this with your predictions in this week's Preview Chart!)

	TARGET	ACTUAL
Timed structured walk (mins)		
Steps		

Abdominal Exercise: ❑

(tick here if you completed your abdominal exercises
today)

date: ———————————

DAY TWENTY

DAILY WALKING TIP: **Hop skip and jump**
To improve balance and co-ordination, build bone and burn fat faster, add some play to your walk. If you walk in a group, break out in a park and play a few minutes of It or Tag! Hop on and off kerbs, zigzag in and out of trees, attack any sloping terrain head on and bunny hop across path edges. Do these moves carefully so you don't trip.

Structured Exercise: ❏

(tick here if you have completed your structured exercise today, then fill in the number of steps and minutes you managed. You can compare this with your predictions in this week's Preview Chart!)

	TARGET	ACTUAL
Timed structured walk (mins)		
Steps		

Abdominal Exercise: ❏

(tick here if you completed your abdominal exercises today)

date: _____

DAY TWENTY ONE

DAILY WALKING TIP: **Wiggle your hips**
Add a race walking hip swivel to increase speed, trim your waistline and burn more calories. Walk slowly, crossing your feet slightly in front of you so one hip rotates forward while the other goes back. Once you get the hang of it, pick up your pace and try it without crossing your feet.

Structured Exercise: ❑

(tick here if you have completed your structured exercise today, then fill in the number of steps and minutes you managed. You can compare this with your predictions in this week's Preview Chart!)

	TARGET	ACTUAL
Timed structured walk (mins)		
Steps		

Abdominal Exercise: ❏

(tick here if you completed your abdominal exercises today)

Weekly Review

END OF WEEK THREE

I took structured exercise on the following days:

	ACTUAL STEPS	ACTUAL MINUTES
M	_____	_____
T	_____	_____
W	_____	_____
T	_____	_____
F	_____	_____
S	_____	_____
S	_____	_____

TOTAL STEPS	TOTAL MINUTES
_____	_____

I did my abdominal exercises on:

M ☐
T ☐
W ☐
T ☐
F ☐
S ☐
S ☐

My measurements:

WEIGHT	WAIST	NAVEL	CHEST	HIPS	THIGH

On reflection my week fell into the following category
(circle the relevant one):

Progressive   **Maintenance**   **Damage
Limitation**

Weekly Preview

START OF WEEK FOUR

Week Four Walking Goals

Walking Novice: 30 minutes continuous walking plus 10,000 steps on your pedometer.

Walking Whiz: 50 minutes continuous walking plus 10,000 steps on your pedometer.

I will take structured exercise on these days:

	TARGET STEPS	TARGET MINUTES
M	_____	_____
T	_____	_____
W	_____	_____
T	_____	_____
F	_____	_____
S	_____	_____
S	_____	_____

	TOTAL STEPS	TOTAL MINUTES
	_____	_____

I will do my abdominal exercises on these days:

M ☐

T ☐

W ☐

T ☐

F ☐

S ☐

S ☐

This week my challenges are:

1. _____

2. _____

3. _____

4. _____

I think the week ahead will fall into the following category (circle the relevant one):

Progressive   **Maintenance**   **Damage Limitation**

date: _____

DAY TWENTY TWO

DAILY WALKING TIP: **Go for a moonwalk**
Put on some reflective clothing, grab your partner or a
friend and a flashlight and head out on a night walk.
Night noises, night stars and even window shopping
can give a refreshing spark to a familiar route. But do
remember to walk in a safe area.

Structured Exercise: ❏

(tick here if you have completed your structured exercise today, then fill in the number of steps and minutes
you managed. You can compare this with your predictions in this week's Preview Chart!)

	TARGET	ACTUAL
Timed structured walk (mins)		
Steps		

Abdominal Exercise: ❏

(tick here if you completed your abdominal exercises today)

date: _____

DAY TWENTY THREE

DAILY WALKING TIP: **Invest in a weighted vest**
Walking with hand weights can strain your shoulders. A safer way to up your intensity is a weighted vest that evenly distributes the extra pounds.

Structured Exercise: ❏

(tick here if you have completed your structured exercise today, then fill in the number of steps and minutes you managed. You can compare this with your predictions in this week's Preview Chart!)

	TARGET	ACTUAL
Timed structured walk (mins)		
Steps		

Abdominal Exercise:　　　❏

(tick here if you completed your abdominal exercises today)

date: ──────────────────

DAY TWENTY FOUR

DAILY WALKING TIP: **Keep up the good work!**
For a double dose of feel good vibes, lend your feet to a cause. Training for and completing a charity walk with a large group of people is exhilarating, and knowing you are ticking off a good deed in the process makes your success all the more enjoyable. In addition, committing to an event will help you keep up your walking programme.

Structured Exercise: ❏

(tick here if you have completed your structured exercise today, then fill in the number of steps and minutes you managed. You can compare this with your predictions in this week's Preview Chart!)

	TARGET	ACTUAL
Timed structured walk (mins)		
Steps		

Abdominal Exercise: ❑

(tick here if you completed your abdominal exercises today)

date: _____

DAY TWENTY FIVE

DAILY WALKING TIP: **Back down**
Walk briskly up a hill or stairs, then slowly go down backwards to stretch the calves, hamstrings and go easy on your knees. Do be careful and watch where you are going.

Structured Exercise: ☐

(tick here if you have completed your structured exercise today, then fill in the number of steps and minutes you managed. You can compare this with your predictions in this week's Preview Chart!)

	TARGET	ACTUAL
Timed structured walk (mins)		
Steps		

Abdominal Exercise: ❑

(tick here if you completed your abdominal exercises today)

date: _____

DAY TWENTY SIX

DAILY WALKING TIP: **Have a coffee break**
Split your walks in two today and plan a route so you
walk to a coffee shop and have a quick coffee and chat
with a friend before completing the second half of your
walk.

Structured Exercise: ☐

(tick here if you have completed your structured exercise today, then fill in the number of steps and minutes
you managed. You can compare this with your predictions in this week's Preview Chart!)

	TARGET	ACTUAL
Timed structured walk (mins)		
Steps		

Abdominal Exercise: ❏

(tick here if you completed your abdominal exercises today)

date: _____

DAY TWENTY SEVEN

DAILY WALKING TIP: **Hit the beach!**
Walking in soft sand boosts your calorie burn by 20–50 %, and it will wake up leg muscles you never knew you had.

Structured Exercise: ❏

(tick here if you have completed your structured exercise today, then fill in the number of steps and minutes you managed. You can compare this with your predictions in this week's Preview Chart!)

	TARGET	ACTUAL
Timed structured walk (mins)		
Steps		

Abdominal Exercise: ❏

(tick here if you completed your abdominal exercises
today)

date: —————————————

DAY TWENTY EIGHT

DAILY WALKING TIP: **Congratulations! You have made it!**
E mail the four friends you contacted at the start of your 28-day programme to tell them you have completed your challenge.

Structured Exercise: ❑

(tick here if you have completed your structured exercise today, then fill in the number of steps and minutes you managed. You can compare this with your predictions in this week's Preview Chart!)

	TARGET	ACTUAL
Timed structured walk (mins)		
Steps		

Abdominal Exercise: ☐

(tick here if you completed your abdominal exercises today)

Weekly Review

END OF WEEK FOUR

I took structured exercise on the following days:

	ACTUAL STEPS	ACTUAL MINUTES
M	_____	_____
T	_____	_____
W	_____	_____
T	_____	_____
F	_____	_____
S	_____	_____
S	_____	_____

	TOTAL STEPS	TOTAL MINUTES
	_____	_____

I did my abdominal exercises on:

M ☐
T ☐
W ☐
T ☐
F ☐
S ☐
S ☐

My measurements:

WEIGHT	WAIST	NAVEL	CHEST	HIPS	THIGH

On reflection my week fell into the following category
(circle the relevant one):

Progressive　　　**Maintenance**　　　**Damage
Limitation**

Monthly Review

END OF THE PROGRAMME!

My weekly step totals:

	TOTAL STEPS	TOTAL MINUTES
Week 1	——————	——————
Week 2	——————	——————
Week 3	——————	——————
Week 4	——————	——————
	GRAND TOTAL STEPS	**GRAND TOTAL MINUTES**
	——————	——————

I did my abdominal exercises on this many days:

_____

My final measurements:

WEIGHT	WAIST	NAVEL	CHEST	HIPS	THIGH

My starting measurements:

WEIGHT	WAIST	NAVEL	CHEST	HIPS	THIGH

Subtracting final from starting measurements, I have lost:

WEIGHT	WAIST	NAVEL	CHEST	HIPS	THIGH

On reflection my month was:
(circle one)

  Inspiring!

Congratulations! You have done a great job – and I hope you enjoyed your 28-day Step Counter Diet. Give yourself a pat on the back!

Be active,

Joanna

Step Counter
Trade Offs

By following the Eating and Exercise Principles behind my Step Counter Diet, you will feel better, have a lot more energy and be trimmer and more toned. The Eating Principles are designed to encourage you to follow a sensible healthy eating plan that is easy to implement at all times – whether at work, at home or out having fun with family and friends. As we all know, the latter can sometimes pose a little bit of a challenge as there are so many tempting things to eat! Life is about enjoying yourself, so my plan is **not** about feeling that you can never have your favourite indulgence. My 80:20 rule and the clever Step Trade Offs are intended to help you keep on track by enjoying a healthier diet that still allows you the odd indulgence!

The 80:20 Rule

The best way to lose weight, body fat and to stay healthy is not to deprive yourself of everything you love, but to stick to the 80:20 rule. With the 80:20 rule the key to successful long-term weight loss is **consistency** rather than being "good" 100% of the time. If you can stick to the Eating Principles 80% of the time, you have succeeded! By being consistent, you can actually eat a little more, you will feel more energized, you will get the results you are seeking and you won't experience the roller coaster of mood swings and lack of energy when you under-eat to "make up" for those "over excesses"!

Step Trade Offs

The aim of the Eating Principles is to help you develop a template for healthy long-term eating that is easy and enjoyable and will improve your health and boost your energy!

To recap, the Eating Principles are:

- Carb Curfew – reduce that bloating
- Frontload Your Day – gain day-long energy
- Stop Portion Distortion – stop excess calories creeping in
- Get Your Calcium – help your body burn fat
- Enjoy the Right Carbs – keep hunger at bay
- Pick the Right Protein – boost your brain power and help you feel satisfied

Applying these principles will automatically help you achieve your daily quota of fruit and veg and a balanced long-term eating plan that works for you. These principles need to form the backbone of your health and body investment – but don't panic – I am not asking you to be a complete saint! Providing you apply the Eating Principles 80% of the time, along with the Step Trade Offs, you can have your indulgences and still remain healthy and keep excess weight-gain at bay.

HOW IT WORKS

Each step you take gives you an average calorie burn. Even when you are not moving, your body is burning calories, using energy to breathe and pump blood around your body in order to carry out all your body's basic daily processes. This is called your resting metabolic rate. Your resting metabolic rate can vary from individual to individual – it is partly genetic and partly depends on your muscle mass. Therefore, we all need to eat a certain number of calories just to carry on living and this is why eating a diet of less than 1000–1200 calories in the long term is not advisable.

We also burn calories when we exercise and increase our daily physical activity levels. These calories are important as they help create our overall Energy Gap. In addition, regular physical activity boosts our health!

Following my Eating Principles with the 28-day walking plan will deliver results. By the end of the 28-day walking plan, you are going to feel so much better and fitter that you probably won't crave those indulgences quite so much – but when you do, you can do a Step Trade Off!

All you need to do is look at the selection of indulgences on the next few pages and see how many steps you need to take to expend the approximate number of calories for each one. I am not saying these are bad foods – rather these foods should be a treat and not a regular daily feature of a healthy diet. It is so simple and everyone wins – you feel you are not being deprived and the additional physical activity will help rev up your metabolism. Your long-term health will improve through regular physical activity.

So with Step Trade Offs you don't have to sacrifice your favourite indulgences – just remember they are an **extra** and not an **everyday** part of your healthy Eating Principles!

Please remember that Step Trade Offs are intended to serve as a guideline only and as such are not definitive. Just as food servings vary in their calorie content, so do people vary in their walking speed and calorie burn rate.

BISCUITS, BREADS, CAKES AND OTHER BAKED GOODS

Serving size 100 grams, unless otherwise stated

Savoury and Sweet Biscuits

Biscotti (Starbucks, 1 biscuit/27g)	100	2500
Chocolate biscuits, full coated	524	13100
Cream crackers	440	11000
Crispbread, rye	321	8025
Digestive biscuits, chocolate	493	12325
Digestive biscuits, plain	471	11775
Gingernut biscuits	456	11400
Oatcakes	441	11025
Rusks, plain	408	10200
Rusks, low sugar	414	10350
Rusks, flavoured	401	10025
Rusks, wholemeal	411	10275
Sandwich biscuits	513	12825
Semi-sweet biscuits	457	11425
Short-sweet biscuits	469	11725
Shortbread	498	12450
Wafer biscuits, filled	535	13375
Water biscuits	440	11000
Wholemeal crackers	413	10325

Large cakes

Battenburg cake	370	9250
Cake mix	331	8275
Cherry cake	394	9850
Chocolate cake	456	11400
Chocolate cake, with butter icing	481	12025
Coconut cake	434	10850
Crispie cakes	464	11600
Fruit cake, rich	341	8525
Fruit cake, rich, retail	322	8050
Fruit cake, rich, iced	356	8900
Fruit cake, wholemeal	363	9075
Gingerbread	379	9475
Lardy cake	375	9375
Madeira cake	393	9825
Sponge cake	459	11475
Sponge cake, fatless	294	7350
Sponge cake, jam filled	302	7550
Sponge cake, with butter icing	490	12250
Swiss roll	276	6900

Small cakes and sweetbreads

Bagel, Cinnamon & Raisin (New York Bagel Co., 1 bagel/85g)	240	6000
Bagel, Onion (New York Bagel Co., 1 bagel/85g)	233	5825
Bagel, Original (New York Bagel Co., 1 bagel/85g)	230	5750
Choux buns	381	9525
Cream horns	435	10875
Crumpets, fresh	177	4425
Crumpets, toasted	199	4975
Currant buns	296	7400
Custard tarts, individual	277	6925
Danish pastries	374	9350
Doughnuts, custard-filled	358	8950
Doughnuts, jam	336	8400
Doughnuts, ring	397	9925
Doughnuts, ring, iced	383	9575
Eclairs, fresh	373	9325
Eclairs, frozen	396	9900
Fancy iced cakes, individual	407	10175
Halva	615	15375
Jam tarts	380	9500
Muffins	283	7075
Muffins, bran	272	6800
Muffin, Classic Blueberry (Starbucks, 1 muffin/129g)	438	10950

Muffin, Skinny Blueberry (Starbucks, 1 muffin/129g)	306	7650
Muffin, Skinny Peach & Raspberry (Starbucks, 1 muffin/120.2g)	286	7150
Rock cakes	396	9900
Rum baba	223	5575
Scones, cheese	363	9075
Scones, fruit	316	7900
Scones, plain	362	9050
Scones, potato	296	7400
Scones, wholemeal	326	8150
Scones, wholemeal, fruit	324	8100
Scotch pancakes	292	7300
Strawberry tartlets	206	5150
Teacakes, fresh	296	7400
Teacakes, toasted	329	8225
Vanilla slices	330	8250
Waffles	334	8350

Sweet and savoury pastries

Cheese pastry, cooked	498	12450
Choux pastry, cooked	325	8125
Flaky pastry, cooked	560	14000
Puff pastry, frozen, raw	373	9325
Samosas, meat	593	14825
Samosas, vegetable	472	11800
Shortcrust pastry, frozen, raw	440	11000

Desserts

Apple pie, one crust	197	4925
Apple pie, pastry top and bottom	266	6650
Arctic roll	200	5000
Blackcurrant pie, pastry top and bottom	262	6550
Bread and butter pudding	160	4000
Cheesecake	411	10275
Cheesecake, Blackcurrant Swirl (Heinz, ⅕ portion/87g)	241	6025
Cheesecake, Chocolate & Hazelnut (Gold Sara Lee, 1 slice/65g)	205	5125
Christmas pudding	291	7275
Flan, pastry, with fruit	118	2950
Flan, sponge, with fruit	112	2800
Flan case, pastry	544	13600
Flan case, sponge	295	7375
Fruit pie, one crust	186	4650
Fruit pie, pastry top and bottom	260	6500
Instant dessert powder	391	9775
Lemon meringue pie	319	7975
Milk puddings	128	3200
Pancakes, sweet	301	7525
Sponge pudding, with dried fruit	331	8275

Sponge pudding, with jam or treacle	333	8325
Sponge pudding, canned	285	7125
Treacle tart	368	9200
Trifle	160	4000
Trifle, with Dream Topping	148	3700
Trifle, with fresh cream	166	4150

CRACKERS, CRISPS, SNACKS AND SNACK BARS

Crackers, Cheese Melts (Carr's, 1 cracker/4g)	19	475
Crisps, New York Cheddar (Kettle Chips, 1 bag/50g)	242	6050
Crisps, Sea Salt with Crushed Black Peppercorns (Kettle Chips, 1 bag/50g)	225	5625
Pringles, Barbecue (1 serving/50g)	267	6675
Pringles, Cheese & Onion (1 serving/50g)	266	6650
Pringles, Original (1 serving/50g)	274	6850
Pringles, Paprika (1 serving/50g)	268	6700
Pringles, Salt & Vinegar (1 serving/50g)	265	6625
Pringles, Sour Cream & Onion (1 serving/50g)	270	6750
Snack Bars, White Chocolate Muesli (Kellogg's Cereal, 1 bar/25g)	110	2750
Snack Bars, Choc Chip (Quaker Harvest Cheweee, 1 bar/22g)	94	2350

Snack Bars, Toffee	94	2350
(Quaker Harvest Cheweee, 1 bar/22g)		
Snack Bars, White Chocolate Chip	94	2350
(Quaker Harvest Cheweee, 1 bar/22g)		
Snack Bars, Apple	130	3250
(Kellogg's Nutri-Grain, 1 bar/37g)		
Snack Bars, Blueberry	130	3250
(Kellogg's Nutri-Grain, 1 bar/37g)		
Snack Bars, Cherry	133	3325
(Kellogg's Nutri-Grain, 1 bar/37g)		
Snack Bars, Chocolate	137	3425
(Kellogg's Nutri-Grain, 1 bar/37g)		
Snack Bars, Elevenses Ginger	170	4250
(Kellogg's Nutri-Grain, 1 bar/45g)		
Snack Bars, Elevenses	162	4050
(Kellogg's Nutri-Grain, 1 bar/45g)		
Snack Bars, Strawberry	133	3325
(Kellogg's Nutri-Grain, 1 bar/37g)		
Snack Bars, Chocolate Caramel	90	2250
(Kellogg's Rice Krispies Squares, 1 bar/21g)		
Snack Bars, Chocolate	74	1850
(Kellogg's Rice Krispies Squares, 1 bar/18g)		

MILK AND MILK PRODUCTS

Serving size 100 grams

Milk and cream

Skimmed milk, average	33	825
Skimmed milk, UHT	32	800
Semi-skimmed milk, average	46	1150
Whole milk, average	66	1650
Whole milk, pasteurised	66	1650
Buttermilk	37	925
Coffee Complement	554	13850
Coffeemate	540	13500
Condensed milk, skimmed, sweetened	267	6675
Condensed milk, whole, sweetened	333	8325
Dried skimmed milk	348	8700
Evaporated milk, whole	151	3775
Flavoured milk	68	1700
Goat's milk, pasteurised	60	1500
Sheep's milk, raw	95	2375
Soya milk, plain	32	800
Soya milk, flavoured	40	1000

Bournvita powder	377	9425
Cocoa powder	312	7800
Drinking chocolate powder	366	9150
Cream, fresh, half	148	3700
Cream, fresh, single	198	4950
Cream, fresh, soured	205	5125
Cream, fresh, whipping	373	9325
Cream, fresh, double	449	11225
Cream, fresh, clotted	586	14650
Cream, UHT, canned spray	309	7725
Dessert Top	291	7275

Cheeses

Cheese, Brie	319	7975
Cheese, Camembert	297	7425
Cheese, Cheddar, average	412	10300
Cheese, Cheddar, English	412	10300
Cheese, Cheddar, vegetarian	425	10625
Cheese, Cheddar-type, reduced fat	261	6525
Cheese spread, plain	276	6900
Cheese spread, flavoured	258	6450
Cottage cheese, plain	98	2450
Cottage cheese, plain, reduced fat	78	1950
Cream cheese	439	10975
Cheese, Danish blue	347	8675
Cheese, Derby	402	10050
Cheese, Edam	333	8325
Cheese, Edam-type, reduced fat	229	5725
Cheese, Emmental	382	9550
Cheese, Feta	250	6250
Fromage frais, plain	113	2825
Fromage frais, fruit	131	3275
Fromage frais, very low fat	58	1450
Full fat soft cheese	313	7825
Goat's milk soft cheese	198	4950
Cheese, Gouda	375	9375

Cheese, Gruyere	409	10225
Cheese, Mozzarella	289	7225
Cheese, Parmesan	452	11300
Processed cheese, plain	330	8250
Processed cheese, smoked	303	7575
Cheese, Ricotta	144	3600
Cheese, Roquefort	375	9375
Soya cheese	319	7975
Cheese, Stilton, blue	411	10275
Cheese, Stilton, white	362	9050

Yoghurts

Whole milk yoghurt, plain	79	1975
Whole milk yoghurt, fruit	105	2625
Whole milk yoghurt, goat's	63	1575
Low fat yoghurt, flavoured	90	2250
Low fat yoghurt, fruit	90	2250
Drinking yoghurt	62	1550
Greek yoghurt, cow's	115	2875
Greek yoghurt, sheep's	106	2650
Soya yoghurt	72	1800

Desserts and Ice Cream

Creme caramel	109	2725
Custard, canned	95	2375
Dream Topping	626	15650
Jelly, made with water	61	1525
Ice Cream, Baileys (Haagen-Dazs, 1oz/28g)	73	1825
Ice Cream, Belgian Chocolate (Haagen-Dazs, 1oz/28g)	89	2225
Ice Cream, Choc Chip Cookie Dough (Ben & Jerry's, 1 serving/100g)	230	5750
Ice Cream, Choc Chip (Haagen-Dazs, 1oz/28g)	80	2000
Ice Cream, Chocolate Fudge Brownie (Ben & Jerry's, 1 serving/100g)	260	6500
Ice Cream, Chocolate Fudge Swirl (Haagen-Dazs, 1oz/28g)	77	1925
Ice Cream, Chocolate Midnight Cookies (Haagen-Dazs, 1oz/28g)	81	2025
Ice Cream, Chunky Monkey (Ben & Jerry's, 1 serving/100g)	280	7000
Ice Cream, Cookies & Cream (Haagen-Dazs, 1oz/28g)	73	1825
Ice Cream, Galaxy (1 bar/60ml)	203	5075
Ice Cream, Honey I'm Home (Ben & Jerry's, 1 serving/100g)	260	6500

Ice Cream, Lemon Pie (Haagen-Dazs, 1oz/28g)	73	1825
Ice Cream, Mars (1 bar/75g)	260	6500
Ice Cream, Pralines & Cream (Haagen-Dazs, 1oz/28g)	77	1925
Ice Cream, Strawberry Cheesecake (Haagen-Dazs, 1oz/28g)	74	1850
Ice Cream, Strawberry (Haagen-Dazs, 1oz/28g)	67	1675
Ice Cream, The Full Vermonty (Ben & Jerry's, 1 serving/100g)	280	7000
Ice Cream, Toffee Crème (Haagen-Dazs, 1oz/28g)	74	1850
Ice Cream, Vanilla Caramel Fudge (Ben & Jerry's, 1 serving/100g)	260	6500
Ice Cream, Vanilla (Haagen-Dazs, 1oz/28g)	70	1750
Mousse, chocolate, rich	178	4450
Rice pudding, canned	89	2225
Sorbet, lemon	131	3275

Dairy-based Sauces and Spreads

Butter	737	18425
Cheese sauce, made with whole milk	197	4925
Cheese sauce, made with semi-skimmed milk	179	4475
Cheese sauce, made with skimmed milk	168	4200
Dairy/fat spread	662	16550
Onion sauce, made with whole milk	99	2475
Onion sauce, made with semi-skimmed milk	86	2150
Onion sauce, made with skimmed milk	77	1925
Margarine	739	18475
White sauce packet mix	355	8875
White sauce packet mix, made up with whole milk	93	2325
White sauce packet mix, made up with semi-skimmed milk	73	1825
White sauce packet mix, made up with skimmed milk	59	1475

READY MEALS AND SIDE DISHES

Baked Beans (Heinz, ½ can/100g)	103	2575
Baked Beans, American (Heinz, 1 serving/130g)	140	3500
Baked Beans, Barbecue (Heinz, ½ can/100g)	82	2050
Baked Beans, Cheezy (Heinz, 1oz/28g)	53	1325
Baked Beans, with Pork Sausages (Heinz, ½ can/207g)	184	4600
Baked Beans, with Vegetable Sausages (Heinz, 1 can/200g)	212	5300
Noodles, Instant Curry (Heinz, 1 serving/85g)	261	6525
Potato, Saute, Deep-Fried (McCain, 1oz/28g)	47	1175
Potato, Saute, Oven-Baked (McCain, 1oz/28g)	56	1400
Potato Skins, Deep-Fried (McCain, 1oz/28g)	52	1300
Potato Smiles, Oven-Baked (McCain, 1oz/28g)	62	1550
Potato Wedges, Chunky (McCain, 10 wedges/175g)	242	6050

Potato Wedges, Spicy (McCain, 1oz/28g)	61	1525
Spaghetti, Bolognese (Heinz, 1 can/400g)	344	8600
Spaghetti, in Tomato Sauce (Heinz, 1 can/400g)	244	6100
Spaghetti, with Sausages (Heinz, 1 can/400g)	328	8200
Spaghetti Hoops, in Tomato Sauce (Heinz, 1 can/400g)	224	5600
Spaghetti Hoops, 'n' Hot Dogs (Heinz, 1 can/400g)	304	7600

SAUCES, DIPS AND DRESSINGS

Serving size 100 grams, unless otherwise stated

Chilli sauce	79	1975
Chutney, mango, sweet	189	4725
Chutney, tomato	128	3200
Cranberry sauce	151	3775
Dressing, French Low-Fat (Hellmann's, 1 tbsp/15g)	9	225
Dressing, French Luxury (Hellmann's, 1 tbsp/15g)	45	1125
Dressing, Garlic & Herb Reduced-Calorie (Hellmann's, 1 tbsp/15ml)	35	875
Dressing, Italian Salad (Hellmann's, 1 serving/50g)	103	2575
Dressing, Orange & Honey Luxury (Hellmann's, 1 serving/15ml)	17	425
Dressing, Salad Light (Heinz, 1 serving/9.8g)	24	600
Hazelnut oil	899	22475
Horseradish sauce (average creamed and plain)	153	3825
Ketchup, BBQ (Heinz, 1 serving/10g)	14	350

Ketchup, Tomato (Heinz, 1 tbsp/15g)	16	400
Ketchup, Wicked Orange (Heinz, 1 serving/11g)	12	300
Mayonnaise, Garlic & Herb Reduced-Calorie (Hellmann's 1 serving/25ml)	58	1450
Mayonnaise (Hellmann's, 1 tsp/11g)	79	1975
Mayonnaise, Light (Hellmann's, 1 serving/10g)	30	750
Mayonnaise, Mediterranean (Hellmann's, 1 tsp/11g)	79	1975
Mayonnaise, Reduced-Calorie (Hellmann's, 1 serving/30g)	90	2250
Pasta Sauce, Basil & Oregano for Bolognese (Ragu, 1 serving/200g)	76	1900
Pasta Sauce, Original for Bolognese (Ragu, 1 jar/525g)	268	6700
Pasta Sauce, Traditional Bolognese (Ragu, 1 jar/515g)	345	8625
Peanut oil	899	22475
Pickle, sweet	141	3525
Redcurrant jelly	240	6000
Relish, burger/chilli/tomato	114	2850
Salad Cream (Heinz, 1 tbsp/10g)	33	825
Salad Cream, Light (Heinz, 1 tbsp/10g)	24	600

Sauce, BBQ Original (Heinz, 1 serving/9.5g)	12	300
Sauce, Curry Medium (Uncle Ben's, 1 serving/100g)	66	1650
Sauce, for Bolognese Light Original (Ragu, 1 jar/515g)	196	4900
Sauce, for Bolognese Original (Ragu, 1 Jar/515g)	242	6050
Sauce, Sweet & Sour Original (Uncle Ben's, 1 pack/300g)	264	6600
Sauce, Sweet & Sour (Uncle Ben's, 1 serving/200g)	168	4200
Sauce, Thai Green Curry Express (Uncle Ben's, 1 pack/170g)	131	3275
Sauce, Tomato Organic (Heinz, 1 tsp/5g)	5	125
Sesame oil	898	22450
Tartare sauce	299	7475
Vinaigrette, Luxury French (Hellmann's, 1 tsp/5ml)	15	375
Walnut oil	899	22475

STORE CUPBOARD ITEMS

Serving size 100 grams, unless otherwise stated

Corn oil	899	22475
Grapeseed	899	22475
Gravy instant granules	462	11550
Molasses	266	6650
Olive oil	899	22475
Popcorn, candied	480	12000
Popcorn, plain	593	14825
Quorn	86	2150
Sugar, brown (average, light and dark)	362	9050
Sugar, white	394	9850
Sunflower oil	899	22475
Stuffing mix, dried	338	8450
Suet, vegetable	836	20900
Stuffing mix, dried, made up	97	2425
Syrup, golden	298	7450
Syrup, golden, pouring	296	7400
Syrup, maple	262	6550
Tomato puree, with salt	76	1900
Tomatoes, sun dried	495	12375
Vegetable oil, blended, average	899	22475
Yeast extract	180	4500

SWEETS AND CHOCOLATE

Chewing Gum, Airwaves (Wrigley's, 1 piece/1g)	2	50
Chewing Gum, Orbit Spearmint (Wrigley's, 1 piece/3g)	6	150
Chocolate, Coconut White (Lindt, 1 square/10g)	61	1525
Chocolate, Dark Orange with Slivered Almonds (Lindt, 1 square/10g)	50	1250
Chocolate, Excellence 85% Cocoa Solids (Lindt, 1 square/8.3g)	44	1100
Chocolate, Ferrero Rocher (Ferrero, 1 chocolate/12.5g)	74	1850
Chocolate, Peppermint Patty (Hershey, 3 patties/41g)	160	4000
Fantasy Mix (Haribo, 1 sm Pack/100g)	360	9000
Horror Mix (Haribo, 1 sm Pack/100g)	360	9000
Kiddies Super Mix (Haribo, 1 pack/100g)	401	10025
Milky Mix (Haribo, 1 pack/175g)	644	16100
American Hard Gums (Haribo, 1 pack/175g)	630	15750
Cola Bottles (Haribo, 1 sm pack/16g)	57	1425

Cola Bottles (Haribo, 1 med pack/175g)	628	15700
Dolly Mixtures (Haribo, 1 pack/175g)	719	17975
Gold Bears (Haribo, 1 pack/100g)	358	8950
Jelly Beans (Haribo, 1 pack/100g)	360	9000
Mint Imperials (Haribo, 1 pack/175g)	695	17375
Starmix (Haribo, 1 pack/100g)	360	9000
Tangfastics (Haribo, 1 pack/100g)	359	8975
Wine Gums (Haribo, 1 pack/175g)	655	16375

DRINKS

Serving size 100 grams, unless otherwise stated

Soft drinks

Appletise 1 glass/200ml	98	2450
Ginger Beer, Classic (Schweppes, 1 can/330ml)	115	2875
Coffee, Caffe Mocha) (Starbucks, 1 tall/200ml	278	6950
Coffee, Frappuccino (Starbucks, 1 serving/454ml)	260	6500
Coffee, Caramel Frappuccino (Starbucks, 1 grande size/473ml)	279	6975
Coffee, Mango Citrus Tea Frappuccino (Starbucks, 1 tall/220ml)	180	4500
Coffee, Strawberries & Cream Frappuccino (Starbucks, 1 serving/ Grande/473ml)	581	14525
Dr Pepper (1 bottle/500ml)	210	5250
Dr Pepper, Diet Soda (1fl oz/30ml)	0	0
Fanta, Lemon (1 can/330ml)	165	4125
Fanta, Light (1 glass/250ml)	5	125
Fanta, Orange (1 can/330ml)	142	3550

Hot Chocolate, with Whipped Cream Grande (Starbucks, 1 grande mug/473ml)	440	11000
Latte, Skimmed Milk (Starbucks, 1 serving/260ml)	88	2200
Latte, Whole Milk (Starbucks, 1 tall/355.2ml)	180	4500
Lucozade, Hydro Active (1fl oz/30ml)	3	75
Lucozade, Orange Energy Drink (1 bottle/500ml)	350	8750
Lucozade, Original (1 sm bottle/345ml)	252	6300
Lucozade, Sport Isotonic Lemon Body Fuel (1 bottle/500ml)	140	3500
Lucozade, Sport Orange (1 bottle/500ml)	140	3500
Lucozade, Tropical (1 bottle/380ml)	266	6650
Red Bull (1 can/250ml)	113	2825
Red Bull, Sugar-Free (1 can/250ml)	8	200
Ribena, Blackcurrant Diluted with Water (1 serving/180ml)	81	2025
Ribena, Light (1 bottle/288ml)	63	1575
Sunny Delight (1 glass/200ml)	88	2200
Sunny Delight, Light (1 glass/200ml)	16	400

Alcohol

Baileys Irish Cream (1 glass/37g)	130	3250
Champagne	76	1900
Lager, alcohol-free	7	175
Lager, low alcohol, average	10	250
Lager, premium	59	1475
Lager, Amstel (1 pint/568ml)	227	5675
Lager, Becks (1 can/275ml)	113	2825
Lager, Budweiser (1 bottle/330ml)	133	3325
Lager, Heineken (1 pint/568ml)	256	6400
Lager, Miller Pilsner (1 bottle/500ml)	150	3750
Lager, Holsten Pils (1 can/440ml)	167	4175
Lager, Stella Artois (1 can/550ml)	222	5550
Red wine	68	1700
Rose wine, medium	71	1775
White wine, dry	66	1650
White wine, medium	74	1850
White wine, sparkling	74	1850
White wine, sweet	94	2350
Port	157	3925
Sherry, dry	116	2900
Sherry, medium	116	2900
Sherry, sweet	136	3400
Spirits, 40% volume (average brandy, gin, rum, whisky and vodka)	222	5550

Recipes

This chapter gives you some ideas for Carb Curfew meals when eating at home, showing you how easy it can be to incorporate the Eating Principles into your life. Following is a collection of recipes for lunchtime and your evening meal. All the recipes are low in fat and calories and provide you with the right balance of nutrients at the right time of the day. The emphasis is on healthy dishes that are easy to cook as well as appetizing and enjoyable to eat.

Lunches

Here is a selection of recipes for your midday meal which provide a good balance of starch and protein. Some you will find work better to eat at home – others can easily be put in a lunch box to go. By omitting some of the starch accompaniments you can also double these up as Carb Curfew dinners.

At the end of each recipe you will see the calorie and fat content per serving.

Mexican-Style Wraps with Beans, Herbs and Vegetables   serves 1

100g canned kidney beans
100g canned asparagus
2 tablespoons plain fromage frais
1–2 tablespoons coriander leaves
1 tablespoon flat-leaf parsley
1 tablespoon finely chopped red onion
1 tablespoon lime juice
1 plum tomato
1 soft flour tortilla
salt and pepper, to taste

In separate sieves, drain the kidney beans and asparagus thoroughly. In a mixing bowl, mash the asparagus until smooth. Stir in the fromage frais, coriander, parsley, onion and lime juice. Season to taste with salt and pepper and set aside.

Quarter the tomato and scoop out the seeds. Cut the flesh into small pieces and fold into the asparagus mixture along with the kidney beans.

Lay a tortilla out on a work surface and spread with the vegetable mixture. Fold over a portion of the left-hand side of the tortilla then roll up from bottom to top to give a cylinder. Eat immediately or wrap in greaseproof paper or kitchen foil and pack in a lunch box.

calories per serving: 293   *fat grams per serving: 10*

Vegetable Menestra   serves 2

150g fresh or frozen peas
150g fresh or frozen broad beans
150g asparagus
1 teaspoon olive oil
1 garlic clove, chopped
25g Serrano ham, chopped
1 teaspoon flour
3 canned artichokes, halved
1 tablespoon chopped fresh parsley

Bring a large saucepan of water to the boil. Add the peas, broad beans and trimmed asparagus, return to the boil and simmer for 3 minutes until the vegetables are cooked but still quite crisp. Drain well.

Heat the oil in a large frying pan and add the chopped garlic. Cook over a medium-low heat, stirring constantly, until the garlic is just golden. Add the ham and cook, stirring, for about 3 minutes, then stir in the flour and cook for another 2–3 minutes.

Stir in the cooked vegetables and artichokes and cook, while stirring, for another 3 minutes until the vegetables are tender and the artichokes are heated through. Transfer to a bowl and sprinkle with the chopped parsley. Serve accompanied by fresh bread or a baked potato, if desired.

calories per serving: 204   *fat grams per serving: 4*

Smoked Chicken and Mexican Black Bean Salad   **serves 2**

150g cooked black beans
40g smoked chicken or turkey
60g red pepper
30g celery, any leaves reserved
15g spring onion
10g fresh coriander
1 teaspoon finely chopped green chilli
juice of 1 lime
salt and pepper, to taste

Place the black beans in a mixing bowl. Cut the smoked chicken or turkey into strips and stir it into the beans. Finely dice the pepper, celery and spring onion and stir them in too.

Roughly chop the reserved celery leaves with the leaves and tender stalks of the coriander. Stir them into the salad with the green chilli. Pour in the lime juice and season to taste with salt and pepper. Transfer to a serving plate or lunch box. Serve with toasted granary bread.

calories per serving: 260   *fat grams per serving: 3*

Salmon, Potato and Asparagus Salad   serves 2

1 large salmon fillet
3 stalks asparagus
150g baby new potatoes
½ mango
50g low-fat yoghurt
½ teaspoon wholegrain mustard
1 tablespoon lemon juice or white wine vinegar
1 tablespoon chopped fresh chives
½ stick celery
140g mixed salad leaves
salt and pepper, to taste

Place the salmon in a shallow pan and cover with water. Bring to the boil, then throw in the asparagus, cover and turn off the heat. Leave to stand until the cooking water reaches room temperature.

Meanwhile, place the potatoes in a large saucepan, cover generously with water and bring to the boil. Lower the heat and simmer for 10 minutes until tender. Drain, refresh under cold running water and set aside to cool.

Chop the mango and combine in a blender with the yoghurt, mustard and lemon juice or vinegar. Process until smooth, then stir in the chives by hand. Season to taste with salt and pepper and place the dressing in the fridge to chill.

Remove the salmon and asparagus from the poaching liquid and pat dry with kitchen paper. Cut both into bite-sized pieces and place in a bowl with the cooled cooked potatoes. Chop the celery finely and add it to the bowl. Gently fold in the mango-yoghurt dressing.

Arrange the mixed salad leaves in a salad bowl, top with the dressed salmon and vegetables and serve.

calories per serving: 285   *fat grams per serving: 13*

Salmon Pizza   serves 1

75g fresh salmon fillet or 200g can pink salmon,
  boned and skinned
1 small pizza base
1–2 tablespoons fresh tomato sauce
1 tomato
1 tablespoon chopped red onion
½ teaspoon dried red chilli flakes (optional)
3 tablespoons low-fat yoghurt
1 sprig fresh dill

Preheat the oven to 220°C/425°F/Gas mark 7. Trim the salmon
of any skin and bones and dice the flesh. Place the pizza base
on a baking tray and spread with the tomato sauce. Dice the
tomato and sprinkle it over the sauce, then sprinkle with the
red onion and chilli flakes. Arrange the diced salmon evenly
over the top.

Bake for 15–20 minutes or until the fish is cooked and the
pizza base is lightly browned. Remove from the oven, spoon on
the yoghurt and garnish with fronds from the sprig of dill.

calories per serving: 365   *fat grams per serving: 18*

Pasta with Spring Vegetables   **serves 1**

100g dried pasta such as penne
1 teaspoon vegetable bouillon powder
50g asparagus spears
50g baby carrots, or sliced regular carrots
50g baby courgettes, or sliced regular courgettes
50g mangetout or fine beans, trimmed
1 teaspoon balsamic vinegar
15g parmesan cheese, shaved
2 teaspoon shredded basil leaves
1 teaspoon finely chopped green part of spring onion
freshly ground black pepper

Bring a large saucepan of water to the boil. Add the vegetable bouillon powder and stir to dissolve. Add the pasta and cook according to the directions on the packet. Leave the pasta to boil while you prepare the vegetables, trimming and slicing them as necessary.

Five minutes before the end of the pasta's cooking time, add the asparagus, carrots, courgettes and mangetout or beans – do not stir. Continue cooking for 5 minutes or until the pasta and vegetables are all al dente. Drain thoroughly.

Place the pasta and vegetables on a serving plate and sprinkle with the balsamic vinegar. Top with the shavings of parmesan, the basil and spring onion. Grind some black pepper over the top and serve.

calories per serving: 229   *fat grams per serving: 7*

Carb Curfew Dinners

Here is a selection of starch-free recipes for your evening meal. You'll find something for every occasion – be it a family dinner, a simple meal for two or a dinner party. The emphasis of the dishes is on protein, essential fats, low-fat dairy products and vegetables. All Carb Curfew dinners also work well as starch-free zone lunches.

At the end of each recipe you will see the calorie and fat content per serving.

Lamb and Vegetable Hot-Pot   **serves 4**

200g onions
200g carrots
200g swede or turnip
200g parsnip
1 tablespoon vegetable oil
500g cubed lamb stewing steak
340ml bitter beer (large can)
1 bay leaf or bouquet garni

Preheat the oven to 150°C/300°F/Gas mark 2. Peel all the vegetables and cut them into bite-sized pieces. In a large non-stick frying pan, heat the oil and add the cubed lamb. Cook over a high heat, stirring frequently until the meat is brown on the outside but not cooked through. Transfer to an oven-proof lidded casserole dish.

Add the vegetable pieces to the frying pan, working in batches if necessary, and cook until just beginning to brown. Transfer the vegetables to the casserole and stir well. Pour in the beer, then add the bay leaf or bouquet garni and season generously with salt and pepper. Cover the casserole and place in the oven for 2 hours. Halfway through the cooking time remove the lid and stir. The hot-pot is done when the meat and vegetables are very tender and most of the beer has been absorbed. Remove the bay leaf or bouquet garni and season to taste before serving.

calories per serving: 424   *fat grams per serving: 15*

Thai Beef Salad   **serves 2**

For the beef:
2 lean beef steaks
juice of 1 lime
1 tablespoon soy sauce

For the salad:
150g tomatoes
100g celery
100g spring onions
100g carrot
15g coriander

For the dressing:
1–2 small red chillies
1 garlic clove
1 teaspoon fish sauce
½ teaspoon palm sugar, brown sugar or honey

Place the steaks in a non-corrosive dish. Set aside 2 table-spoons of the lime juice in a small bowl and pour the remainder over the steaks. Add the soy sauce to the meat and set aside to marinate for 30–60 minutes.

Meanwhile, make the salad. Using a small knife, score a cross in the base of each tomato. Place them in a heat-proof bowl and cover with boiling water. Leave to stand for 1–2 minutes, then drain and refresh under cold water. When cool, peel and core the tomatoes. Discard the seeds and cut the flesh into strips. De-string the celery and cut into matchsticks. Cut the spring onions into fine strips. Use a vegetable peeler to cut the carrot into ribbons. Combine the vegetables in a salad bowl. Roughly chop the coriander, including the tender stalks, and stir it into the vegetables.

To make the salad dressing, crush the chillies and garlic together using a pestle and mortar to make a paste. Stir in the reserved 2 tablespoons of lime juice, plus the fish sauce and sugar or honey.

Heat a griddle over a very high heat for about 5 minutes or until very hot and smoking. Add the marinated steaks and immediately turn the heat down to medium-low. Cook for 1–2 minutes on each side, depending on how thoroughly you like steak cooked.

Pour the salad dressing over the vegetables and toss well. Place the vegetables on serving plates and top with the cooked steak – you can cut the steak into strips first if you prefer.

calories per serving: 444   *fat grams per serving: 19*

Gammon Steaks with Thai-Style Salsa   serves 2

2 x 125g gammon steaks
Vegetable oil spray

For the salsa:
100g tomatoes
100g cucumber
100g carrots
50g celery
50g spring onions
1 tablespoon chopped fresh coriander
6 tablespoons lime or lemon juice
1–2 teaspoons fish sauce or soy sauce, to taste
4 tablespoons mild sweet chilli sauce

First make the salsa. Chop all the vegetables very finely and place in a bowl. Stir in the remaining ingredients and set aside to marinate while you cook the gammon steaks.

Heat a griddle or heavy-based frying pan over a very high heat. Spritz the pan with vegetable oil spray, then lay the gammon steaks in the pan and lower the heat to medium. Cook for about 3 minutes on each side until nicely browned and hot.

Serve the gammon steaks immediately with the salsa.

calories per serving: 291   *fat grams per serving: 10*

Chicken and Apricot Tagine   **serves 4**

8 skinless, boneless chicken thighs
150g dried apricots, chopped
225g onions, chopped
225g mushrooms, chopped
725ml chicken or vegetable stock
a pinch of saffron
a pinch of ginger
a pinch of cumin
salt and pepper, to taste
fresh coriander to garnish (optional)

Place all the ingredients in a large, heavy-based saucepan or casserole dish and bring to the boil. Cover, lower the heat right down and simmer for 45 minutes, stirring occasionally.

When cooked, remove the lid and simmer uncovered until most of the liquid evaporates and you have a thick stew. Adjust the seasoning to taste and serve garnished with fresh coriander if desired.

calories per serving: 259   *fat grams per serving: 5*

Light Chicken Curry with Spinach   serves 2

2 medium-large onions, finely chopped
500ml chicken or vegetable stock
1 large Bramley or other cooking apple, peeled, cored and diced
1 tablespoon sultanas
1 heaped tablespoon garam masala
2 part-boned chicken breasts
140g baby spinach leaves
fresh coriander to garnish
salt and pepper, to taste
a little freshly grated nutmeg (optional)

Place the onions and half the stock in a casserole dish or heavy-based saucepan and bring to a hard boil. Lower the heat, cover and leave to simmer for 15 minutes until the onions are tender. Remove the lid and raise the heat a little. Simmer until the liquid has almost evaporated, then add the apples and sultanas and cook for 5 minutes, stirring occasionally. Add the garam masala and stir to give a thick sauce, then add the chicken and stir until thoroughly coated with the sauce. Pour in the remaining stock and bring to the boil. Cover and lower the heat right down so that the stew simmers very gently for 30 minutes.

Uncover the stew and remove the cooked chicken to a plate. Raise the heat under the pan and simmer until the sauce mixture has reduced to a thick coating consistency. Return the chicken to the pan and add salt and pepper to taste. Allow to heat through briefly.

Meanwhile, place the washed spinach in a large saucepan over a low heat. Cover and cook for 5 minutes, stirring occasionally, until the leaves have wilted. Add salt and pepper to taste, plus some grated nutmeg if desired.

Divide the spinach between the serving plates. Top with the chicken and sauce and garnish with the fresh coriander.

calories per serving: 402   *fat grams per serving: 9*

Swedish Chicken and Apple Salad   **serves 2**

For the salad:

175g ready-cooked chicken breast, diced
1 small dessert apple, cored and sliced
1 carrot, coarsely grated
2 spring onions, sliced
15g walnut pieces, chopped
1 small head chicory leaves
salt and freshly ground black pepper, to taste
salad cress, to garnish

For the dressing:

100ml low-fat plain yoghurt
½ teaspoon mild curry paste
1 tablespoon fresh lemon juice
1 small garlic clove, crushed
½ teaspoon sugar
3 tablespoons freshly chopped herbs (eg. parsley, mint and dill)
salt and freshly ground black pepper, to taste

Blend all the dressing ingredients together in a small bowl. Add the diced chicken, sliced apple, carrot, spring onions and walnuts. Season well. Mix together and then chill for 30 minutes.

To serve, line a serving platter with the chicory leaves and pile the salad on top. Scatter the salad cress over the dish and serve.

calories per serving: 292   *fat grams per serving: 9*

Salmon, Cannellini and Lemon-Infused Stew

serves 2

225g salmon fillet, skinned and cut into 2.5cm cubes
2 lemons
½ tablespoon olive oil
1 small onion, finely chopped
1 celery stick, finely chopped
2 bay leaves
227g can tomatoes
275ml vegetable stock
salt and pepper, to taste
227g can cannellini beans
chopped fresh parsley to garnish

Grate the rind of one lemon and shred a few strips from the other. Squeeze the juice of both and put aside.

Heat the oil in a large pan, add the onion and celery and fry for 10 minutes until softened. Stir in the bay leaves, tomatoes and stock. Season and simmer, uncovered, for 20 minutes.

Stir in the lemon juice and grated lemon rind, beans and salmon. Simmer for 8–10 minutes until the salmon is cooked. Spoon the stew into bowls and garnish with the lemon-rind strips and parsley.

calories per serving: 314   *fat grams per serving: 13*

Grilled Hake with Mushroom and Sweetcorn Sauce   serves 2

2 x 150g hake fillets (haddock, cod or skate works well too)
1 heaped teaspoon cornflour
140ml fish stock
20ml low-fat double cream
50g button mushrooms, finely sliced
2 egg yolks
1 small can sweetcorn, drained
olive oil spray
chopped fresh dill, to garnish

Mix the cornflour with a little water to make a smooth paste. Stir into the fish stock on a low heat and add the cream.

Dry-fry the sliced mushrooms. Gently heat the egg yolks in a bowl immersed in a pan of boiling water, adding a few drops of water as needed to create a smooth paste. Stir this into the fish stock and then add the mushrooms and sweetcorn.

Spray the fish with the olive oil and grill for about 5 minutes until brown, turning regularly.

To serve, place the fish on serving plates, top with the sauce and garnish with dill. This dish is lovely served with a fresh green salad.

calories per serving: 362   *fat grams per serving: 11*

Poached Oriental Seabass with Cucumber, Ginger and Spring Onion   **serves 4**

4 x 100g seabass fillets
1 teaspoon coconut milk
25g enoki (strand) or baby button mushrooms
½ teaspoon sesame oil
1 tablespoon lime juice
6 sprigs fresh coriander
2 tablespoons soy sauce
salt and freshly ground black pepper

For the garnish:
15g ginger, shredded
25g spring onion, shredded
25g cucumber, shredded

Place the coconut milk, mushrooms, sesame oil, lime juice, coriander and soy sauce in a shallow pan with 900ml of water. Bring to a simmer without a lid.

Season the fish and place in the water; poach gently. Remove the fish and keep warm. Increase the heat and reduce the poaching liquid by half. Pour the liquid over the fish and garnish with the remaining ingredients.

calories per serving: 168   *fat grams per serving: 5*

Spanish White Bean Stew   serves 2

800g cooked or canned white beans such as cannellini or
   butter beans
1 large green pepper
1 large onion
1 large tomato
1 large carrot
1 red or green chilli
vegetable stock, to cover
2 teaspoons olive oil
salt and pepper, to taste

Finely dice all the vegetables. Place in a large saucepan with the drained beans. Stir, then add enough vegetable stock to cover the ingredients. Bring to the boil over a high heat, then lower the heat right down and cover. Simmer for 30 minutes or until the stew is soft, stirring occasionally. Season to taste with salt and pepper. Divide amongst serving bowls and drizzle each bowl with 1 teaspoon olive oil before serving.

calories per serving: 383   *fat grams per serving: 8*

Steamed Tofu and Aubergines with Aromatic Chinese Sauce   **serves 2**

220g plain or smoked tofu
200g aubergine
100g asparagus
100g broccoli

For the sauce:
2 tablespoons soy sauce
2 teaspoons oyster-flavoured sauce
2 teaspoons chilli sauce
2 teaspoons sesame oil
2 spring onions, chopped

Cut the tofu into equal-sized cubes. Finely slice the aubergine and cut the asparagus and broccoli into bite-sized pieces. Fill a saucepan with water to a depth of about 2$^{1}/_{2}$ cm and place a steamer over the top. Bring the water to the boil. Lay the tofu in the steamer and surround it with the aubergine, broccoli and asparagus. Cover and steam for 5 minutes.

In a small saucepan, combine the soy sauce, oyster sauce, chilli sauce and sesame oil. Bring to the boil and simmer for 2–3 minutes or until the mixture has thickened slightly.

Use a fish slice to transfer the cooked tofu and vegetables to serving plates. Pour the hot sauce over the top and garnish with the chopped spring onions.

calories per serving: 127   *fat grams per serving: 11*

Pumpkin and Mushroom Stew   serves 4

1 large pumpkin, about 30cm diameter
200g onions
200g mushrooms
2 tablespoons olive oil
300ml vegetable stock
6 tablespoons flaked almonds or pine kernels
3 tablespoons low-fat fromage frais
2 tablespoons chopped fresh parsley
salt and pepper, to taste

Peel, core and deseed the pumpkin. Cut the flesh into bite-size pieces. Slice the onions and mushrooms. Heat the oil in a very large saucepan. Add the onions and stir-fry until golden. Add the pumpkin and continue cooking, stirring frequently, until it begins to brown. Add the mushrooms and cook until they begin to soften. Pour the vegetable stock into the pan, bring to the boil, then lower the heat and simmer until the pumpkin is tender and the cooking liquid has evaporated.

Meanwhile, in a dry frying pan, toast the almonds or pine kernels over a moderate heat, stirring frequently, until golden brown. Remove to a plate to cool.

When the pumpkin is tender, remove the pan from the heat and stir in the fromage frais and parsley. Generously season to taste and serve scattered with the toasted nuts.

calories per serving: 348   *fat grams per serving: 30*

Cheesey Baked Bean Hot-Pot   **serves 2**

450g canned baked beans in tomato sauce
225g canned chopped tomatoes
100g green or red pepper, finely chopped
2 teaspoons ready-made crispy onions
2 teaspoons chopped chives
2 tablespoons vegetarian Worcestershire-style sauce or brown sauce
20g grated low-fat Cheddar cheese
100g spinach leaves
pinch grated nutmeg
salt and pepper, to taste

In a small saucepan, place the baked beans, pepper, crispy onions, chives, Worcestershire sauce and cheese. Heat gently, stirring frequently, until the cheese has melted and the other ingredients are hot and tender. Season to taste.

Meanwhile, rinse the spinach leaves, shake dry and put them in a large saucepan with a pinch of salt. Cover and cook over a moderate heat for 3–5 minutes until the spinach has wilted.

Remove the lid, raise the heat and add the nutmeg. Cook, stirring often, until the juices have evaporated from the pan and the spinach is relatively dry. Season to taste. Arrange a bed of spinach on a serving plate and top with the cheesey baked beans.

calories per serving: 279   *fat grams per serving: 6*

Pedometer User Information

FEATURES

1. Counts number of steps up to maximum of 99999.
2. Press white **RESET** key to zero counter.

POWER

1. Powered by 1 x 1.5V DC (AG13) battery.
2. To maintain accurate readings, battery should
   be changed every 12 months.

TECHNICAL DATA

1. Operating temperature range: −5°C to +40°C.
2. Pedometer is accurate to $\pm$ 5%.
3. Pedometer will not record steps accurately if
   used whilst running, walking very quickly or jumping.
4. To ensure accurate readings, clip pedometer firmly to
   waistband (see illustration). **Position pedometer carefully**
   so you are not likely to hit reset button accidentally when
   in use.
5. Care should be taken when removing and inserting
   batteries in battery compartment.